Neurosonological Evaluation of Cerebral Venous Outflow

Giovanni Malferrari
Marialuisa Zedde
Patrizio Prati

Neurosonological Evaluation of Cerebral Venous Outflow

An Ultrasound Atlas

Springer

Giovanni Malferrari
Marialuisa Zedde
Stroke Unit, Neurology Unit,
Dept. of Neuromotor Physiology
Arcispedale Santa Maria Nuova IRCCS
Reggio Emilia
Italy

Patrizio Prati
CIDIMU
Torino
Italy

Videos to this book can be accessed at http://www.springerimages.com/videos/978-88-470-5465-3

ISBN 978-88-470-3936-0 ISBN 978-88-470-5465-3 (eBook)
DOI 10.1007/978-88-470-5465-3
Springer Milan Heidelberg New York Dordrecht London

Printed on acid-free paper

Springer is part of Springer Science+Business Media (www.springer.com)

Foreword

Although the physiological mechanisms associated with cerebral-venous outflow are poorly understood, abnormalities of the venous system have been implicated in a variety of neurological disorders, including multiple sclerosis. This has raised intriguing questions about how to best evaluate the involvement of the venous system in those disorders.

In 2009, it was proposed that abnormalities of the venous system called chronic cerebrospinal venous insufficiency (CCSVI) could be the cause or one of the causes of multiple sclerosis. In late 2010, the Italian Multiple Sclerosis Foundation funded a large Italian multicenter observational study (CoSMo) to evaluate the association between CCSVI and multiple sclerosis. Its results and confirming findings by different studies recently published do not support the role of CCSVI as a recognizable clinical condition that is causally related to the development or progression of MS. The rigorous ultrasound technology and methodology adopted in the CoSMo study was instrumental to provide a clear answer to people with and affected by multiple sclerosis. The Italian neurosonology societies (Società Italiana di NeuroSonologia ed Emodinamica, SINSEC, chaired by Dr Massimo Del Sette and Società Interdisciplinare Neurovascolare, SINV, chaired by Dr Giovanni Malferrari) together with Prof. Erwin Stolz, Department of Neurology, Justus-Liebig-Universität, Giessen, Germany, and the 26 trained sonologists distributed overall in Italy, played a key role in the CoSMo study.

In this book, Giovanni Malferrari, Maria Luisa Zedde, and Patrizio Prati present a comprehensive description of advanced Ultrasound and Imaging Fusion technologies to assess the abnormalities of the venous system in neurological diseases. The Italian Multiple Sclerosis Foundation, who supported the publishing of this book, believes that it will certainly contribute to further educate at the optimum use of these technologies toward the correct diagnosis of abnormalities of the venous system and management of patients.

November 2013

Mario Alberto Battaglia
University of Siena, Italy

Contents

Abbreviations

ACA	Anterior cerebral artery
ACC	Anterior condylar confluent
AJV	Anterior jugular vein
AVM	Artero-venous malformation
BCV	Brachiocephalic vein
BVR	Basal vein of rosenthal
CCA	Common carotid artery
CS	Cavernous sinus
CSA	Cross-sectional area
CTA	Computed tomography angiography
dMCV	Deep middle cerebral vein
ECA	External carotid artery
EJV	External jugular vein
FAV	Artero-venous fistula
GV	Galen vein
ICA	Internal carotid artery
ICV	Internal cerebral vein
IJV	Internal jugular vein
IPS	Inferior petrosal sinus
ISS	Inferior sagittal sinus
MCA	Middle cerebral artery
MRI	Magnetic resonance imaging
PCA	Posterior cerebral artery
PRF	Pulse repetition frequency
SPaS	Sphenoparietal sinus
SPS	Superior petrosal sinus
SRS	Straight sinus
SSS	Superior sagittal sinus
SV	Subclavian vein
SVC	Superior vena cava
SyS	Sigmoid sinus
TBI	Traumatic brain injury
TCCS	Transcranial color-coded duplex sonography
TCD	Transcranial doppler
TS	Transverse sinus
VA	Vertebral artery
VV	Vertebral vein

Part I
Extracranial veins

1 Ultrasound Machine: The Significance of Venous Preset

The study of cerebral venous hemodynamics can be properly carried out by using any ultrasound machine belonging to the last or next-to-last generation, paying adequate attention to adapting the main technical parameters of the machine to the characteristics of the circle to be assessed.

In particular, as regards the extracranial veins, the first element to be taken into account is the probe. In fact, concerning the B-mode frequency range, there are no substantial changes compared to the study of the corresponding arterial bed (carotid and vertebral arteries). Frequencies between 5 and 10 MHz are usually employed, depending on the thickness and size of the neck's soft tissues.

Sometimes it can be difficult to explore the valvular and subvalvular segments of the internal jugular vein (IJV) by using a linear probe. Therefore, the most challenging segments are the confluence between IJV and the brachiocephalic vein (BCV) and similarly the end of the vertebral vein (VV). In such cases, it is possible to overcome this problem by using a trapezoidal steering with the linear probe or by using a micro-convex probe. In the latest case, there is, however, the drawback of greater spatial distortion of the insonated structures than by using the linear probe.

The examination may be carried out not only in fundamental harmonic, but also in harmonic imaging (mainly second harmonic), with 5–7 MHz emission frequency for the more superficial district, that is most of the course of the IJV, and 3–5 MHz for the deeper one (proximal jugular and vertebral veins). With appropriate time gain compensation, the harmonic imaging may allow to maximize the signal-to-noise ratio, thus making it easier to detect morphological changes, spontaneous echo contrast and valve leaflets motility abnormalities, as well as any partial or complete intraluminal content, also thrombotic one.

In order to adjust the color-mode settings, the peculiarities of the venous circulation must be taken into account, i.e., the blood flow velocity, which is relatively lower compared to the corresponding arteries, and the characteristics of the venous flow waveform. In fact, especially in the proximity of the right atrium, during the cardiac cycle, the venous flow may present an alternation of directions with a precise encoding, which is evaluable via an adequate pulse repetition frequency (PRF). Similarly, it is possible to assess the presence of phasic reflux, linked to the breath cycle, at the valvular plane. As for the B-mode, the use of the automatic trapezoidal steering allows to achieve a wider view and to reliably judge the flow direction of the main

Electronic supplementary material Supplementary material is available in the online version of this chapter at http://dx.doi.org/10.1007/978-88-470-5465-3_1. Videos can also be accessed at http://www.springerimages.com/videos/978-88-470-5465-3

G. Malferrari et al., *Neurosonological Evaluation of Cerebral Venous Outflow*,
DOI: 10.1007/978-88-470-5465-3_1, © Springer-Verlag Italia 2014

veins and the corresponding arteries. The most used frequencies range from 3 to 6 MHz, depending on the depth of the structures to be explored. The PRF must be adapted on the basis of the flow velocity. The ranges from the VV to the IJV are usually from 0.5 to 2 kHz in the supine position and from 2 to 0.5 kHz in the sitting position.

The sampling of the Doppler waveform can be and must be obtained in all the explored venous segments, preferably by enlarging the size of the sample volume to cover the entire diameter of the vessel. Also, in this case the more informative frequency is around 3 MHz and the PRF must be adapted on the basis of the velocity values of each segment.

Throughout the examination, it is necessary to bear in mind that even minimal skin compression can alter the size and flow of the veins, since they are easily compressible by the application of a small transluminal gradient. Therefore, the probe must be placed on the skin with a sufficient amount of gel, but without making a direct pressure on the same, except when one wants to verify the absence of thrombotic processes within the IJV.

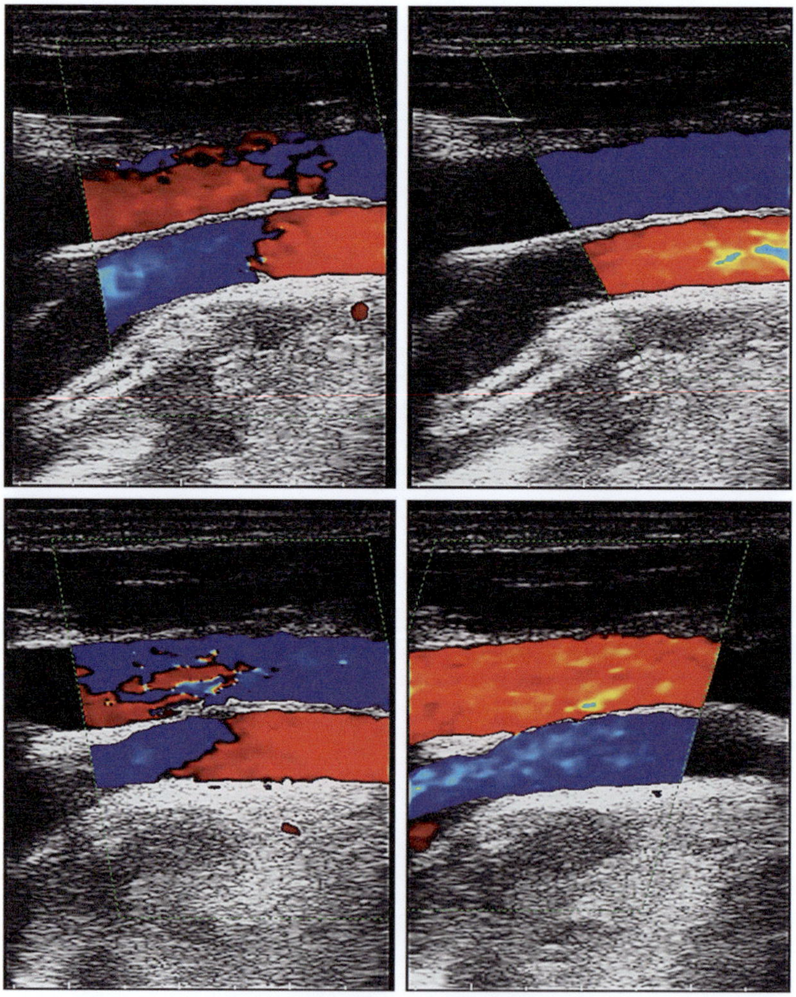

Fig. 1.1 IJV in longitudinal scanning plane. The B-mode has no steering, and the color box has a variable degree and direction of steering. Therefore, there is a different visualization of color filling and flow direction in the same vessel. The more angled *left* and *right* steering makes possible a better visualization of vein to artery relation and relative flow direction changes

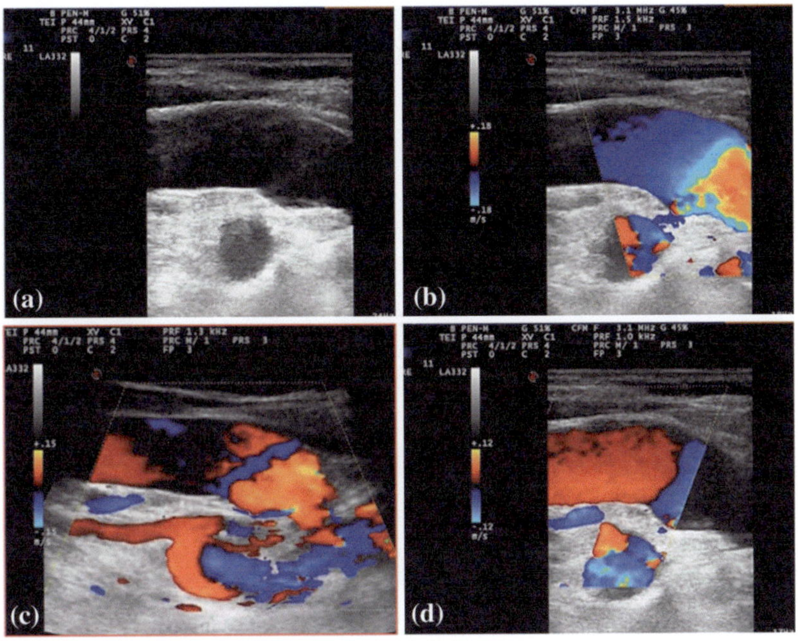

Fig. 1.2 J1 IJV in longitudinal scanning plane with steering. The role of steering both for B-mode and for color mode is crucial at the valve level, because of the lesser possibilities of probe tilting at the base of the neck. **a** B-mode without steering at the valve level. **b** Color box right steering. **c** Color box left steering. **d** B-mode and color box trapezoidal steering: The field of view is markedly increased with a reliable panoramic view. A dynamic evaluation of these examples is illustrated in Movie 1.1

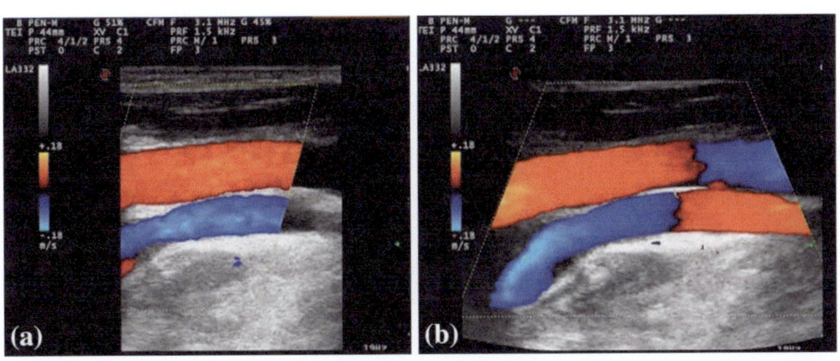

Fig. 1.3 J2 IJV in longitudinal scanning plane. **a** B-mode without steering and color box with *left* steering. **b** B-mode and color box with trapezoidal steering. Without moving the probe with trapezoidal steering, a larger panoramic view is possible

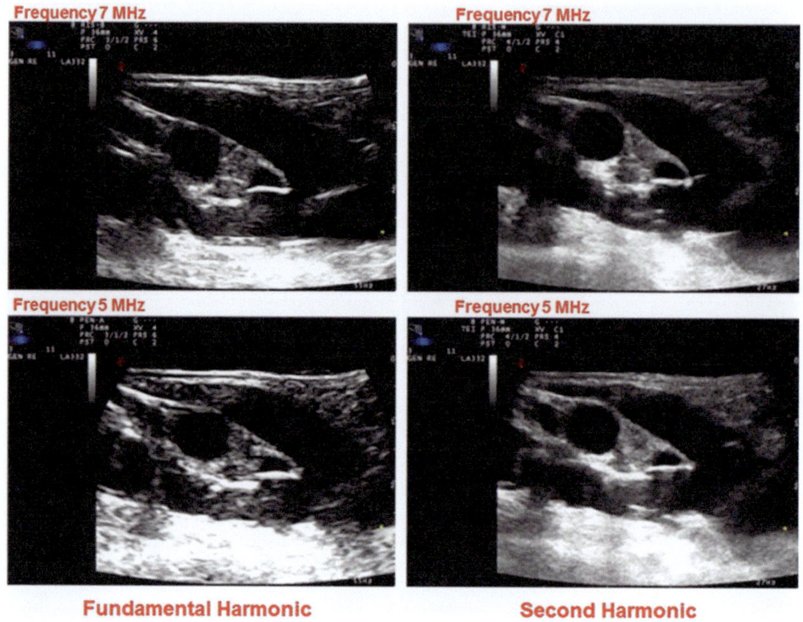

Fig. 1.4 J1 IJV in longitudinal scanning plane. B-mode frequency. An example of the frequency-dependent ultrasound imaging at J1 IJV in longitudinal scanning plane. In this example, two frequencies have been used in B-mode, 7 MHz and 5 MHz, both in fundamental harmonic imaging (*left column*) and in second harmonic (*right column*) imaging. In fundamental harmonic imaging, the decrease in insonation frequency causes a less detailed reconstruction, because of the superficial level of IJV; in second harmonic imaging, there is not a significant loss of quality, while decreasing frequency. A dynamic example is illustrated in Movie 1.2

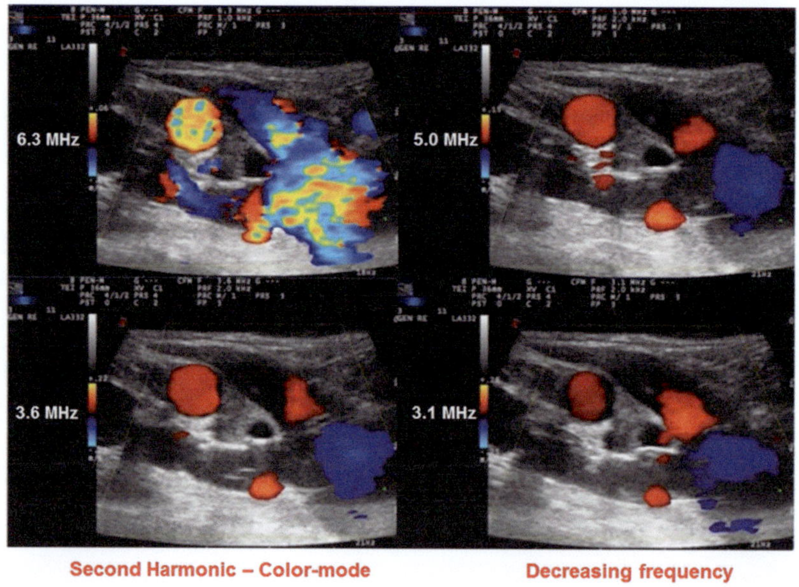

Fig. 1.5 J1 IJV in longitudinal scanning plane. B-mode and color-mode frequency. Another example of the frequency-dependent ultrasound imaging is at J1 IJV in longitudinal scanning plane and second harmonic imaging, at 6.5 MHz central frequency in B-mode. In this example, four frequencies have been used in B-mode: 6.3, 5, 3.6, and 3.1 MHz. With the decrease in color-mode frequency, there is also a decrease in color filling in IJV and VV. A dynamic example is illustrated in the Movie 1.3

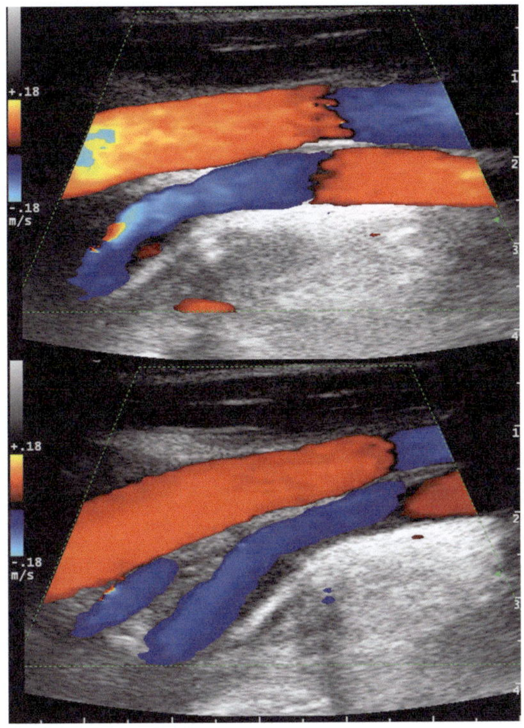

Fig. 1.6 Trapezoidal steering. Example of trapezoidal steering in the evaluation of IJV in the longitudinal scanning plane (Movie 1.4). In both images, at J2 level and at J3 level, the flow direction inversion points in the venous and in the arterial pathways can be easily identified with a specular pattern between IJV and common carotid artery (CCA)

2 Ultrasound Anatomy and How to do the Examination

Most of the cerebral venous drainage is carried by the extracranial venous system in the neck. The main routes of drainage are the IJVs, the vertebral venous system, and the deep cervical veins, presenting a wide inter-individual variability both in the functional prevalence between them and in the postural effect [1–5].

These three routes of cerebral venous outflow have their multiple anastomoses in the neck, especially in the craniocervical junction [1, 3]. The IJV and VV can be easily identified and dynamically studied with ultrasound technique.

2.1 Jugular Veins

IJV is the vein of greater size in the cervical region and is considered the main cerebral venous outflow route, particularly in the supine position. The cerebral venous flow goes mainly from the superficial and deep venous system to the transverse sinus (TS) which in its turn continues in the sigmoid sinus (SyS), which drains into the IJV. The IJV joins the subclavian vein (SV) to form the BCV. The confluence of the two brachiocephalic veins gives rise to the superior vena cava (SVC), which drains the cerebral venous blood in the right atrium.

The IJV therefore begins at the level of the jugular foramen, after the junction of the inferior petrosal sinus (IPS) with the SyS, as a direct continuation of the latter. At this level, there is a slight expansion, called jugular bulb or gulf, which cannot be explored by ultrasound, and which continues relying on the anterior surface of the transverse process of the atlas [6]. The interaction between these two structures may obstruct the jugular venous outflow in some cases evidenced by neurosurgery. However, not even this segment can be investigated by ultrasound, while the next segment, at the level of epistropheus or C2, becomes explorable. In this segment, the relationships of contiguity of the IJV with the carotid axis are easily recognizable. The most common course of IJV is slightly anterior and lateral compared to the internal carotid artery (ICA), with a distance of about 1 mm from it in 69.5 % of examined cases. Variations in the anatomy of the IJV and its correlation to CCA are frequent [7]. The subsequent course of the IJV maintains this relationship with CCA, passing under the anterior edge of the sternocleidomastoid muscle to join the SV and converge into the BCV [8].

In a study performed with computed tomography angiography (CTA) aimed to evaluate the IJV anatomy and its relationship to

Electronic supplementary material Supplementary material is available in the online version of this chapter at http://dx.doi.org/10.1007/978-88-470-5465-3_2. Videos can also be accessed at http://www.springerimages.com/videos/978-88-470-5465-3

G. Malferrari et al., *Neurosonological Evaluation of Cerebral Venous Outflow*,
DOI: 10.1007/978-88-470-5465-3_2, © Springer-Verlag Italia 2014

the carotid artery, out of 176 IJV examined both from the right and from the left side compared to the CCA, 85.2 % of IJV were in a lateral position, 12.5 % in the anterior position, 1.1 % in the medial position, and 1.1 % in the posterior position [7]. Furthermore, in an ultrasonic study designed to evaluate the degree of overlap between the IJV and CCA in the position of the head suitable for IJV cannulation, in over 1,000 veins, the IJV covers even if only partially the CCA in 54 % of patients, predisposing them to the accidental puncture of the carotid artery [9]. The variability may be even greater if you consider the effect of the rotation of the head; in fact, the overlap between IJV and CCA increases passing from the neutral position of the head to a rightward rotation (23.3 vs. 39.2 %) and to a leftward one (35.3 vs. 52.8 %), so that the incidence of lateral positioning of the IJV compared to the CCA is significantly reduced with the rotation of the head (40 vs. 21 % at right, 26.5 vs. 10.5 % at left). The right side appears, however, associated with a minor overlap, whatever the position of the head [10].

An important and well-studied element of the IJV is its valve apparatus, located near the confluence with the SV, and present in 86–93 % of the veins in autopsy case studies [11].

From the ultrasound point of view, it is therefore possible to divide the IJV into three different segments:

- a rostral segment or J3, bounded below by the carotid bifurcation and corresponding to the IJV segment before receiving the confluence of the common facial vein.
- an intermediate segment or J2, between the carotid bifurcation and the supravalvular plan,
- a lower segment or J1, consisting of the valve plane and of the dilation immediately supravalvular.

Morphological anatomical abnormalities of IJV are considered rare; for example, duplication would have a ratio of 4/1000 unilateral cervical dissections [12].

2.2 Internal Jugular Vein Valves

The high-resolution ultrasound examination revealed the presence of a valve in one or both veins in 87 % of cases in the series of Lepori et al. [13] and in 72 % in the series of Macchi and Catini [14]; the series of Darge et al. [15] in a population of children and young adults has found instead a prevalence of 96 %. In autoptic studies on adults, the 86–88 % of the examined subjects had a valve [16, 17]. Gender differences in the prevalence of the valvular apparatus of the IJV are not reported, and in the subjects with unilateral valve, it is more commonly located to the right side.

Murase et al. [18] in an autoptic study judged as competent 88 % of the valves located on the right side and only 44 % of those located on the left one. Furthermore, it is known that the cerebral venous drainage is asymmetric, with the right side more frequently dominant than the left one. From these findings, it can be hypothesized that the dominant side is more frequently equipped with a valve.

The valve cusps are macroscopically described in anatomical studies as thin translucent structures; the majority of valves are composed of two cusps (66–90 %). Monocusp valves are the second most common form, while tricusp valves account for 6–7 % [15].

The valves are located on the distal portion of the IJV (J1, in the ultrasound subdivision above suggested), proximal to the jugular bulb [13]. Physiologically, a complete closure of the valve occurs during diastole, in order to prevent the retrograde transmission of the right atrial pressure through the SVC and BCV into the IJV [19].

2.3 Size of the IJV and Cross-Sectional Area

There is a broad range of normality regarding the size (in terms of cross-sectional area—CSA) and the symmetry of the IJV. The limits of the information available in the literature depend on the fact that most of the published studies have not been performed on normal subjects but on intensive care units patients, with the aim of evaluating the options and risks of a jugular venous catheterization. They are often hypo- or hypervolemic subjects with hemodynamic and respiratory diseases, thus making the data difficult to be exported to normal subjects. Furthermore, in the context of neuroradiological studies, for example CTA, there is not the possibility to assess the influence of breath dynamics on the IJV CSA. Under these restrictions, there are some ultrasonic studies that show, at the J2 level, how the normal venous diameter may vary from 9.1 to 10.2 mm, although a much smaller IJV, with diameter less than 5 mm, according to the evaluation of the authors, can be found in 13.5 % of the subjects on the right side and in 10.6 % on the left one [20]. In this category of patients, that is subjects with kidney disease for whom central venous catheterization was required so as to obtain access for dialysis, the angiographic study also indicated the presence of anatomical abnormalities of the central veins (IJV, SCV, BCV), including stenosis and/or angles, especially in those with a previous history of jugular catheterization with tunneled catheters (65 vs. 30 %) [21].

The use of CT angiography for the measurement of the diameter of the IJV bilaterally showed that 80.5 % of people have a dominant size of the right IJV [22, 23]. Furthermore, 7/176 IJV have been identified as hypoplastic, and in one case, such a condition was present bilaterally [22]. These considerations led the authors to suggest the priority of the right side for central venous catheterization.

Also for the IJV diameter, as well as for the presence of valves, there are no differences in gender and age [24].

The factors that can affect the size of the IJV are many, including the conditions of hydration, the cardiac and respiratory situation, which determine the intrathoracic pressure, the position of the head, and extrinsic compression by other structures in the neck, owing to the high compressibility of the venous vessels for the low pressures within them [25]. Some positional maneuvers, such as the controlateral head rotation, may result in an increase in the area of the IJV examined with a consensual reduction in contralateral vein area, almost an occlusion. Similar increase in the area can be determined by the position of Trendelenburg [26, 27].

Another condition that can affect the area of the IJV is the occurrence of a phlebectasia, which is a focal dilatation of the terminal bulb of the IJV in the immediately subvalvular area; it is a benign condition, most frequently found in pediatric patients because it determines the appearance of a mass of the lower cervical region, most common on the right side for a more direct transmission of the intrathoracic pressure through the shortest innominate vein, also potentially equipped with valves [28, 29]. The ultrasound appearance of jugular phlebectasia is that of a fusiform dilation of the vessel, which, after execution of Valsalva maneuver, has a further considerable increase in size, both compared to the values of healthy control subjects and when compared to the contralateral IJV. The ratio of the diameter of the IJV at rest/Valsalva was calculated in 1:22 in normal subjects and 1:72 in patients [29].

2.4 Branches of the IJV

There are several venous branches that drain into the IJV in its cervical course. Among these, in the rostro-caudal direction, the most important are the facial vein, the lingual, the superior and middle thyroid veins. The first three can join in various ways, forming the thyreo-linguo-facial trunk, which is called facial or thyreo-facial vein before draining into the IJV. In addition, the main branches of the IJV of the two sides are connected by several midline anastomotic branches, helping to maintain an adequate venous outflow. Also, IJV branches are provided with valves, as demonstrated by an anatomical study [30]. The frequency (number of valves/cm of course) is variable: 0.24 ± 0.16 in the facial vein, 0.07 ± 0.15 in the lingual vein, $0.05 \pm$

0.10 in the superior thyroid vein, and 0.22 ± 0.40 in the media thyroid vein.

When the valves are present, they may be continent, thereby preventing retrograde venous flow, or incontinent, thus forming part of the circuit of regurgitation in case of retrograde transmission of venous hypertension [31].

The branches of the IJV may be identified by ultrasound, both in transverse scan and in longitudinal scan, B-mode and color mode, and similarly also the Doppler waveform can be sampled. During the cross-sectional scanning of the jugular axis, it is frequently possible to identify the terminal portion of IJV branches, as tributaries thereof, usually at the level of the cervical medium segment either J2 and J3 or rostral (submandibular), less frequently at the caudal level, J1 segment. The Valsalva maneuver often facilitates the identification of the IJV branches, as well as allowing the identification of possible valve incontinence of the same or of the circuits of regurgitation. Once the branches of the IJV have been identified in this way, the transition to a longitudinal scan allows to follow a segment of greater length and also to identify the outflow into the IJV or the presence of any valves, as described also by some studies [32]. In longitudinal scanning, both in color mode and in Doppler mode, it is possible to identify the flow direction of a single branch of the IJV, as well as to apply the Valsalva maneuver to identify a possible reflux.

2.5 Superficial Veins of the Neck

The superficial veins of the neck and head are highly variable with a few fixed elements:

- The superficial temporal vein and the maxillary vein join to form the retromandibular vein, which branches as it crosses the parotid. The posterior branch, together with the posterior auricular vein, forms the external jugular vein (EJV), whereas the anterior branch joins the facial vein to form the common facial vein which flows into the IJV. The EJV crosses the sternocleidomastoid muscle in the superficial fascia, passes through the roof of the rear triangle, and then pierces the deep fascia 2.5 cm above the clavicle to connect either in the confluence between IJV and SV (60 %), or in the SV (36 %), or in the IJV (4 %). It is not rarely duplicated [33]. Also, the EJV presents the valves, usually two, one in the end portion, near the confluence, and one approximately 4 cm above the level of the clavicle [34].

The anterior jugular vein (AJV) originates at the level of the hyoid bone from the confluence of blood from the superficial veins, from the branches of the EJV, from facial veins or from the same IJV. It runs alongside the neck midline, crossing the thyroid isthmus. It connects with the contralateral vein (jugular arc) just above the sternum, and subsequently, it deepens and flows into the SV (54 %) or into the EJV (46 %) [35]. There is sometimes the possibility of a single AJV in the midline instead of two peer structures [36].

2.6 Vertebral Veins

The vertebral venous system forms a network of vessels freely communicating, without valves either transverse or longitudinal. It consists of an inner part, the intraspinal epidural venous plexus, and of an outer part, paravertebral plexus, both of which continue for the entire length of the spinal cord. The system communicates with the deep thoracic and lumbar veins, the intercostals veins, the azygos and hemiazygos veins, as well as with the inferior vena cava.

The vertebral venous system presents a rather complex organization, since it is mainly constituted by two elements, the vertebral venous plexus and the VV (i.e., the venous plexus of the vertebral artery—VA) [3, 37, 38]. The vertebral venous plexus can be subdivided into an internal plexus (internal vertebral plexus, anterior and posterior) and an outer plexus (external vertebral plexus, anterior and posterior).

The VVs are the main longitudinal part of the external vertebral venous system. The VVs and the deep cervical veins, which are located within the muscle layers of the neck, receive flow from the marginal sinus and SyS through the condylar veins and their emissaries and from the venous plexus surrounding the foramen magnum. In addition, there are several segmental connections between the internal and external parts of the vertebral venous system. The VVs, the deep cervical veins, and the EJV join the BCV.

The deep cervical veins and the VVs are considered to be the external component of the vertebral venous plexus. The intervertebral veins connect the VVs with the internal vertebral venous plexus within the spinal canal [39]. The VV exits the transverse foramen at the level of C7 as a single trunk, which flows into the back side of the BCV.

The complex connections of the vertebral venous outflow with the vertebral venous system at the skull cervical junction have been demonstrated both in anatomical and in angiographic studies [3, 41]. Among these, the most important and unvarying structure is the anterior condylar confluent (ACC), into which the lateral and anterior condylar veins, the IPS, and the IJV flow. The numerous anastomoses of the ACC make it an intersection between the cavernous sinus (CS), the dural sinuses of the posterior fossa, and the cervical posterior outflow tract (vertebral venous system and deep cervical veins).

The posterior and lateral condylar veins allow the connection with the external vertebral venous plexus, whereas the anterior condylar veins are linked to the internal vertebral venous plexus. There are anastomoses between the anterior external vertebral venous plexus, the VVs, and the deep cervical veins located in the region of the craniocervical junction.

The pterygoid plexus and the facial veins are other important ways of side extracranial outflow.

The pterygoid plexus communicates with the CS and finally drains into the EJV [37]. The facial vein can receive the venous flow from the superior ophthalmic vein, which reverses when the venous pressure in the CS is high [42, 43].

2.7 Doppler Waveform

The IJV and the VV have a largely similar Doppler waveform since they are affected by analogous hemodynamic parameters. However, the morphology of the Doppler waveform of the IJV is described in greater detail.

The heart contractions and the changes in the intrathoracic pressure are reflected in the Doppler waveform. During expiration or the Valsalva maneuver, the intrathoracic pressure increases, leading to a reduction in the venous return and to an increase in the diameter of the IJV. In this phase, we observe a poor or absent flow. During inspiration, the venous flow is increased as a result of negative intrathoracic pressure, and this produces a waveform of greater amplitude.

The typical Doppler waves, S, v, D, and a, at the level of the SCV can usually be identified also in the J1 segment of the IJV.

The normal venous flow is influenced by the retrograde pulsatility determined by cardiac movements and phasic changes associated with breathing.

The respiratory phase in the venous waveform depends on many factors, including the distance of the vein from the thorax. The venous spectrogram includes the S waves, v, D and a:

S: systolic wave, determined by the negative intra-atrial pressure with the movement of the atrioventricular septum toward the cardiac apex

v: is the result of the intra-atrial positive pressure created by overdistension of the right atrium during the filling phase.

D: diastolic wave determined by the negative intra-atrial pressure, consequence of the opening of the tricuspid valve

a: reflects the intra-atrial positive pressure during the atrial.

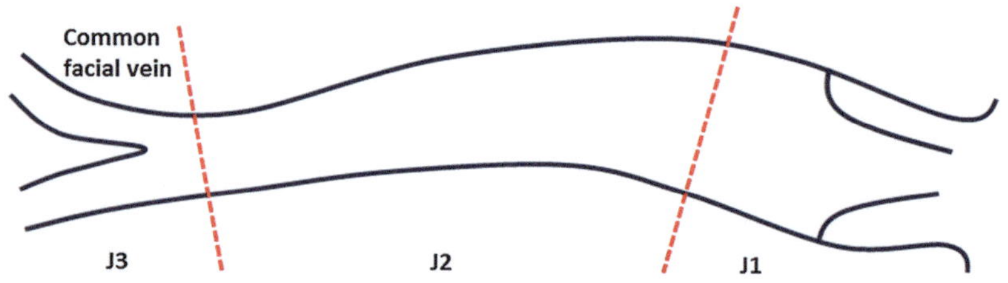

Fig. 2.1 Schematic drawing of IJV and its segments. J1 or proximal segment, focused to the valve system. J2 or intermediate segment. J3 or distal segment, where the common facial vein ends into the IJV

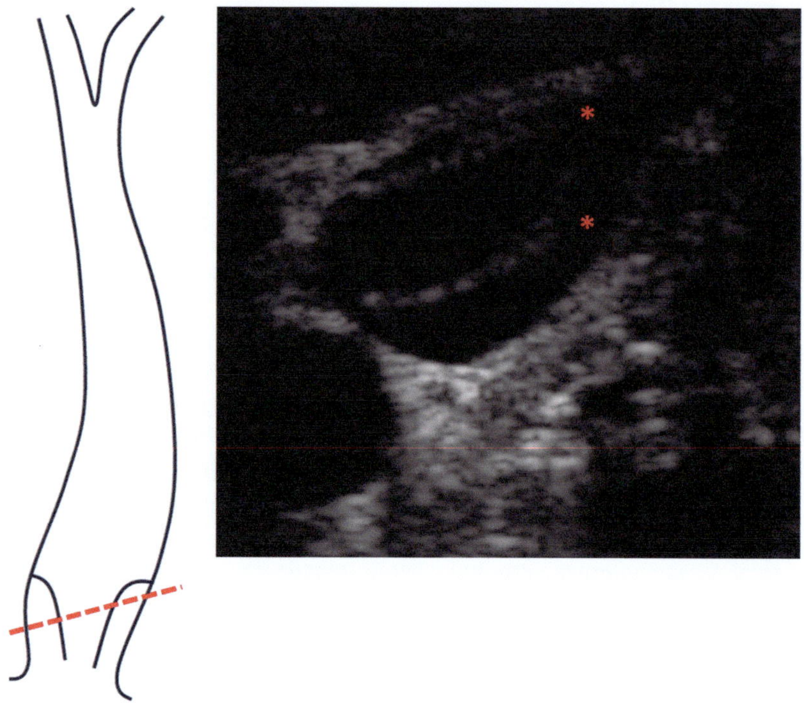

Fig. 2.2 IJV in transverse scan at the level of the valve leaflets (J1) in B-mode. The valve system is well identifiable with two cusps in an intermediate position between the complete opening and the closure. The valve leaflets (see the *asterisks*) seem as *hyperechoic curve* and *tiny lines* coming from one side to the other of the vessel wall within the lumen. Movie 2.1 shows a dynamic example of the leaflets' movement

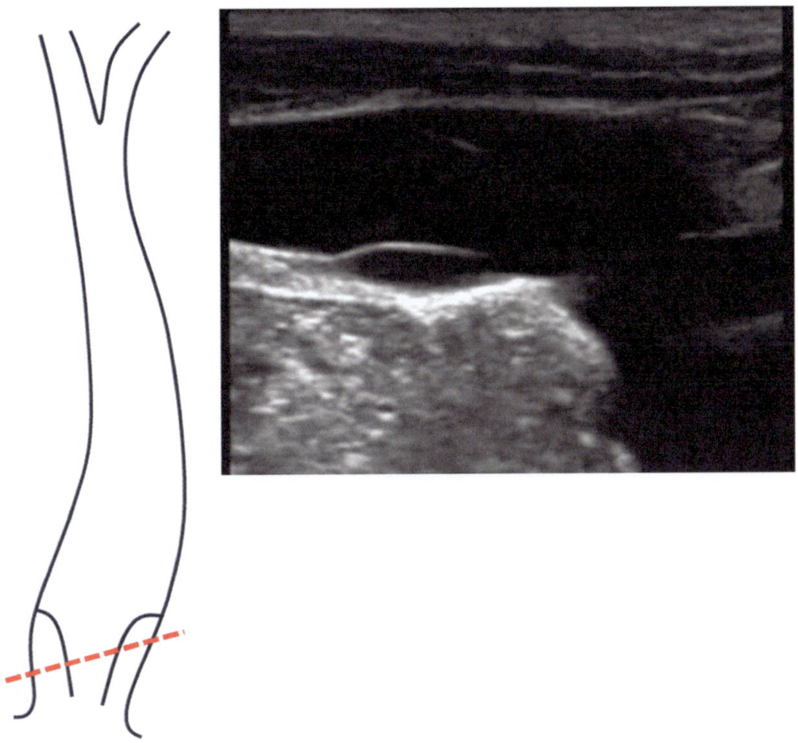

Fig. 2.3 Longitudinal scan of the IJV at the level of the valve system (J1) in B-mode. Also in this case are well evident the valve leaflets as two slightly *hyperechoic lines* into the IJV lumen, stopped in an intermediate position during the opening–closing cycle. The valve cusps define the valve sinuses (*white asterisks*) at the IJV bulb. Movie 2.2 shows a dynamically view of the leaflets movement

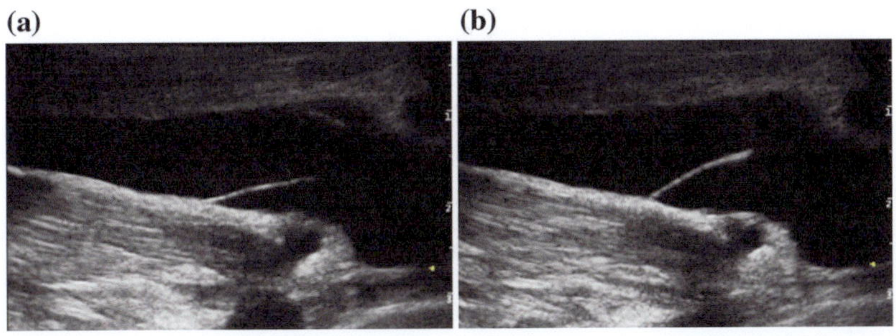

Fig. 2.4 Longitudinal scan of IJV at the valve level (J1) in B-mode, focusing on a particular aspect. In the *left side* **a,** the valve is totally open and has two well-identifiable separate leaflets; in the *right side* **b,** the valve is close and the leaflets are adherent each to other into the IJV lumen near the *midline*. Pictures are oriented leaving the head of the examined subject on the *left* end and the heart on the *right* end

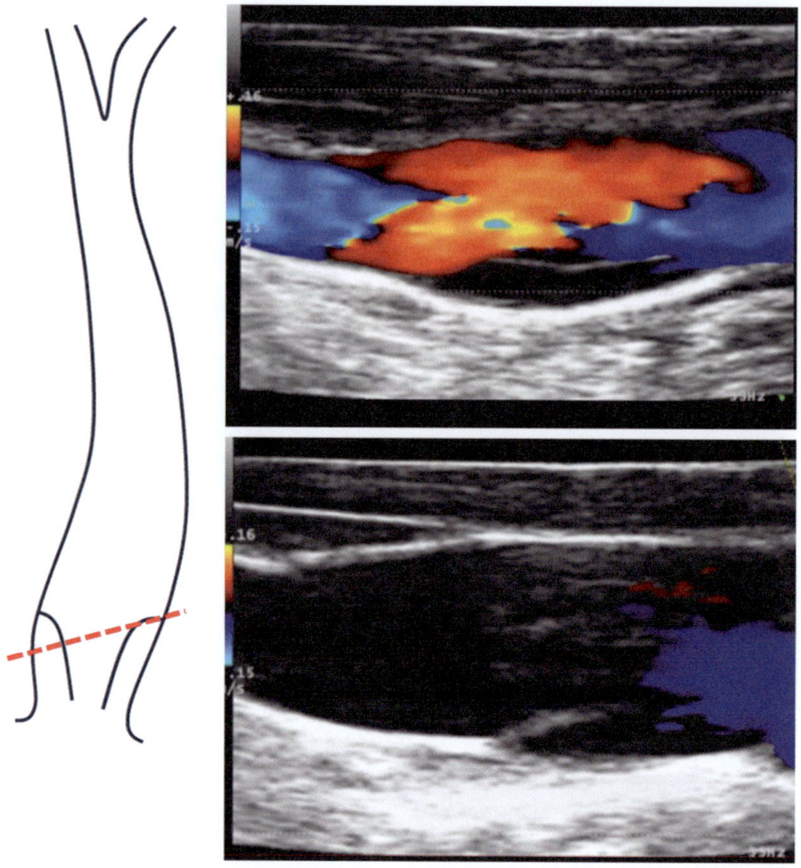

Fig. 2.5 Longitudinal scan of IJV at the valve level (J1) in color mode; the subject is the same as in Fig. 2.4. In the *left side* of the picture, there is the schematic drawing of the IJV with the level of insonation. In the *right side*, the two magnified pictures show the color-coded signal of blood flowing through the open valve (*top image*) and the stopped color-coded signal of blood flow because of the valve closure. The pictures are oriented as detailed in the caption of the Fig. 2.4

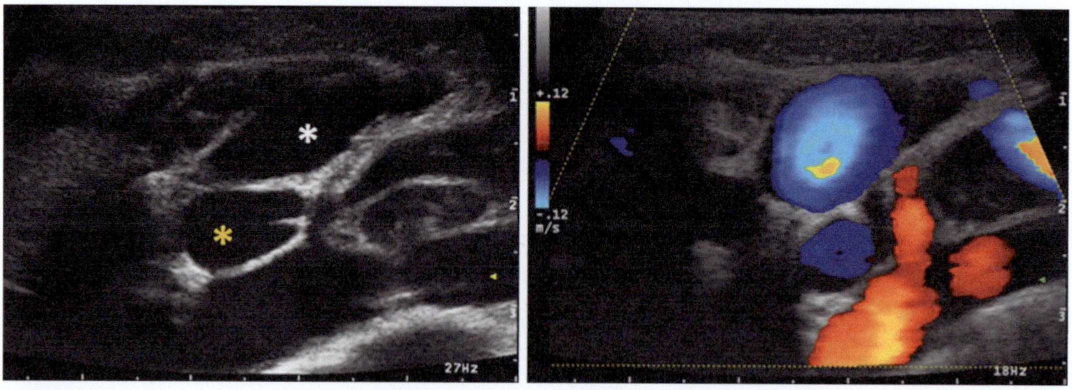

Fig. 2.6 Transverse scan of J1 IJV in B-mode (in the *left side*) and in color mode (in the *right side*). It is often possible to simultaneously visualize the IJV and VV valve system, as in present picture is exemplified. IJV (*white asterisk*) and VV (*yellow asterisk*) are imaged in the same picture at the level of the valve system of both veins, See also the correspondent Movies 2.3 and 2.4

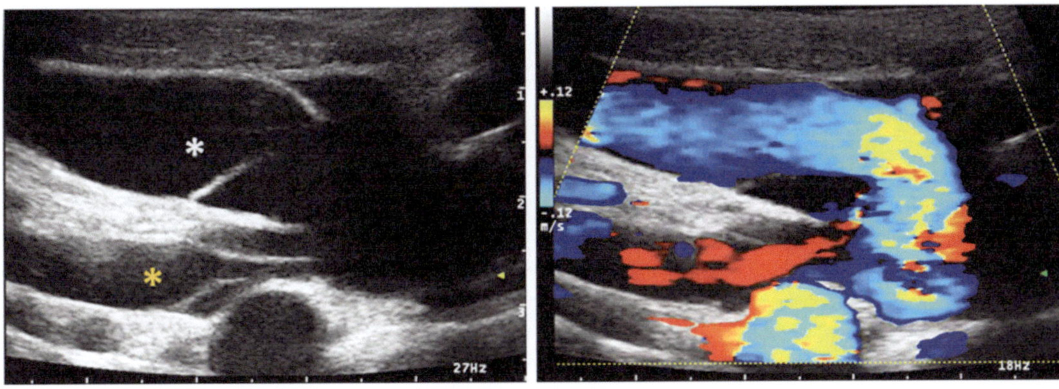

Fig. 2.7 Longitudinal scan of J1 IJV in B-mode (in the *left side*) and in color mode (in the *right side*). As in the Fig. 2.6, it is often possible to simultaneously visualize the IJV and VV valve system, as in present picture is exemplified in longitudinal scan. IJV (*white asterisk*) and VV (*yellow asterisk*) are imaged at the valve level. The valve system seems composed from two leaflets for both veins. See also the correspondent Movie 2.5

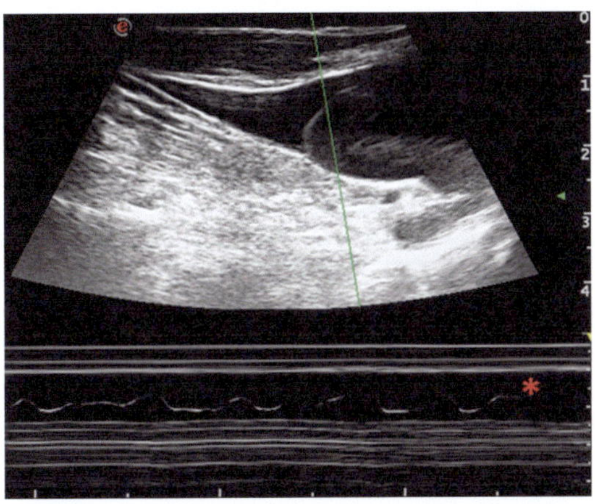

Fig. 2.8 Longitudinal scan of IJV at the valve level (J1) in M-mode. Another way of evaluate the valve leaflets movement is by using M-mode as echocardiographic evaluation of valve function. The M-mode allows to evaluate the movement of the structures at different depth levels along the sampling line (*M-line*). The *M-line* in the picture is *green*, and, in the lower part of the image, the *asterisk* indicates the *line* correspondent to the cycles of movement of one IJV leaflet. See also the Movie 2.6

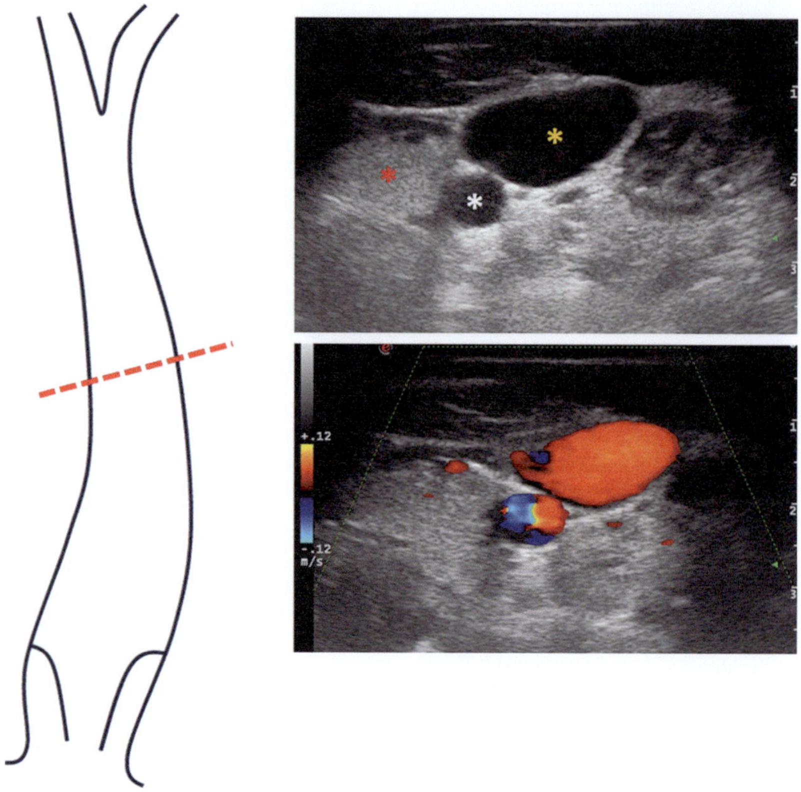

Fig. 2.9 Transverse scan of IJV at the level of the thyroid gland (J2) in B-mode (*upper part* of the picture) and in color mode (*lower part* of the picture). The *red asterisk* indicates the thyroid gland, the *white* one the common carotid artery, and the *yellow* one indicates the IJV

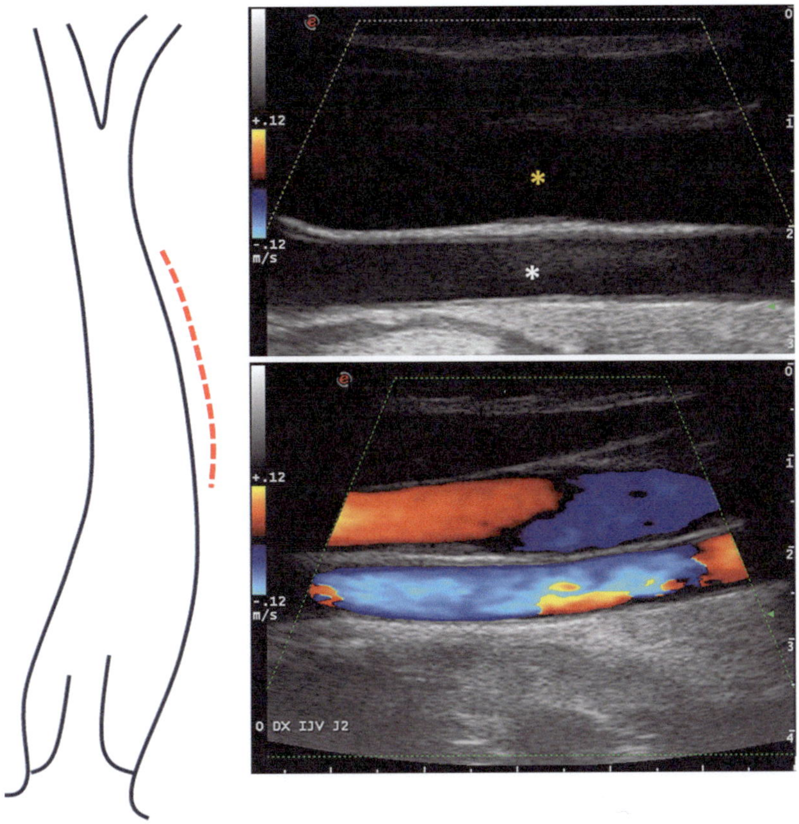

Fig. 2.10 Longitudinal scan of IJV at the level of the intermediate segment (J2), in B-mode (*upper part* of the picture) and in color mode (*lower part* of the picture). The *white asterisk* indicates the CCA and the *yellow* one the IJV, and upon the IJV course, the suprafacial muscular planes of the neck are identifiable. In this example, IJV is parallel to the CCA within the same sheath and both vessels are visible in the same scanning plane but with opposite blood flow direction, as shown in color mode. See also the correspondent Movie 2.7

(a)

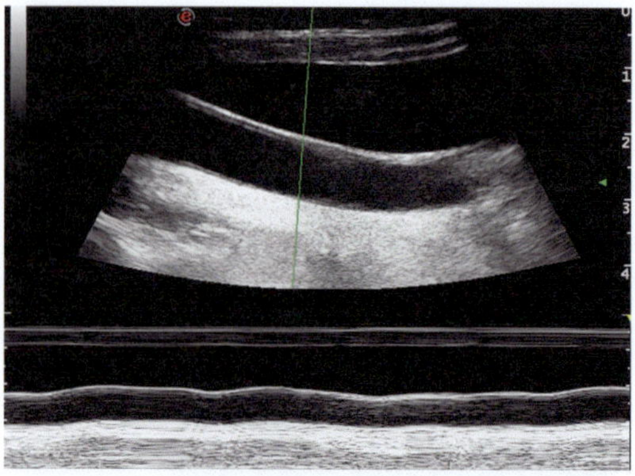

(b)

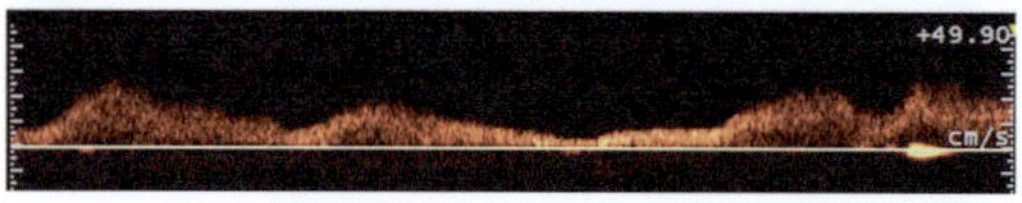

Fig. 2.11 **a** Longitudinal scan of IJV at the level of the intermediate segment (J2) in M-mode. By using this scanning mode, it is possible to evaluate the width of the movement of expansion–contraction of the IJV in comparison with the movements of the CCA, as reference for the heart cycle. It is noticeable that the variations in the IJV diameter are different in each heart cycle because of the superimposed effect of the breath cycle. It is sometimes difficult to differentiate one component from the other one, especially in some situations, as in the presence of IJV valve incontinence or pulmonary hypertension, where the breath-dependent variations can be much more accentuated. **b** This variability is expressed in the Doppler waveform that is affected by the same components, as in this example

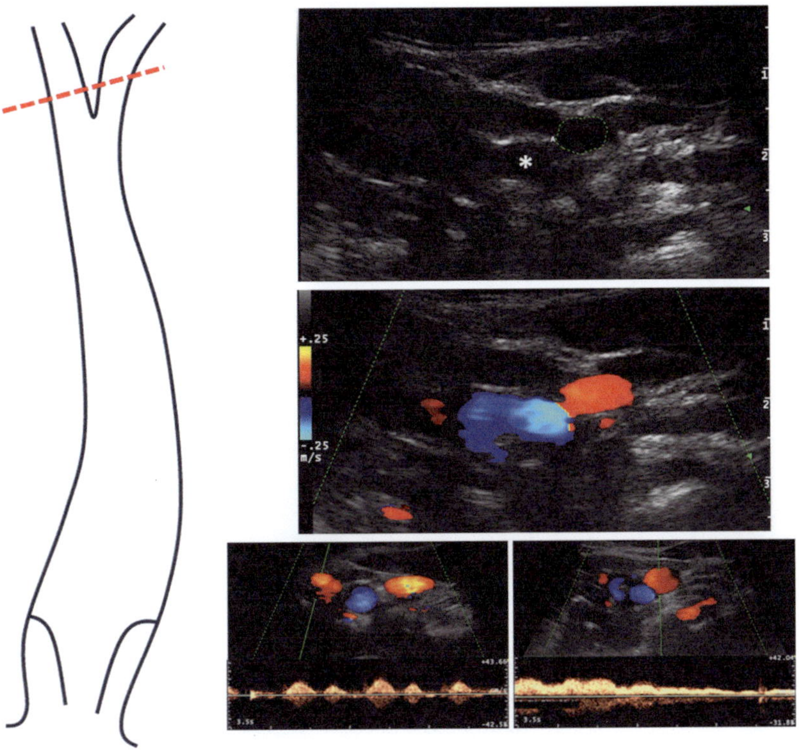

Fig. 2.12 Transverse scan of IJV at the level of the distal segment (J3) in B-mode and color mode. From up to bottom: (1) image in B-mode with manual tracking of J3 IJV CSA; on the *left side* (*white asterisk*), there are the CCA and the external carotid artery (ECA), slightly upon the carotid bifurcation, and besides there is the common facial vein (see also the Movie 2.8). (2) Image in color mode of the same structures with the opposite direction of blood flow in arteries and veins showed by Doppler waveform. (3) Doppler waveform of the common facial vein (*left side*) and J3 IJV (*right side*)

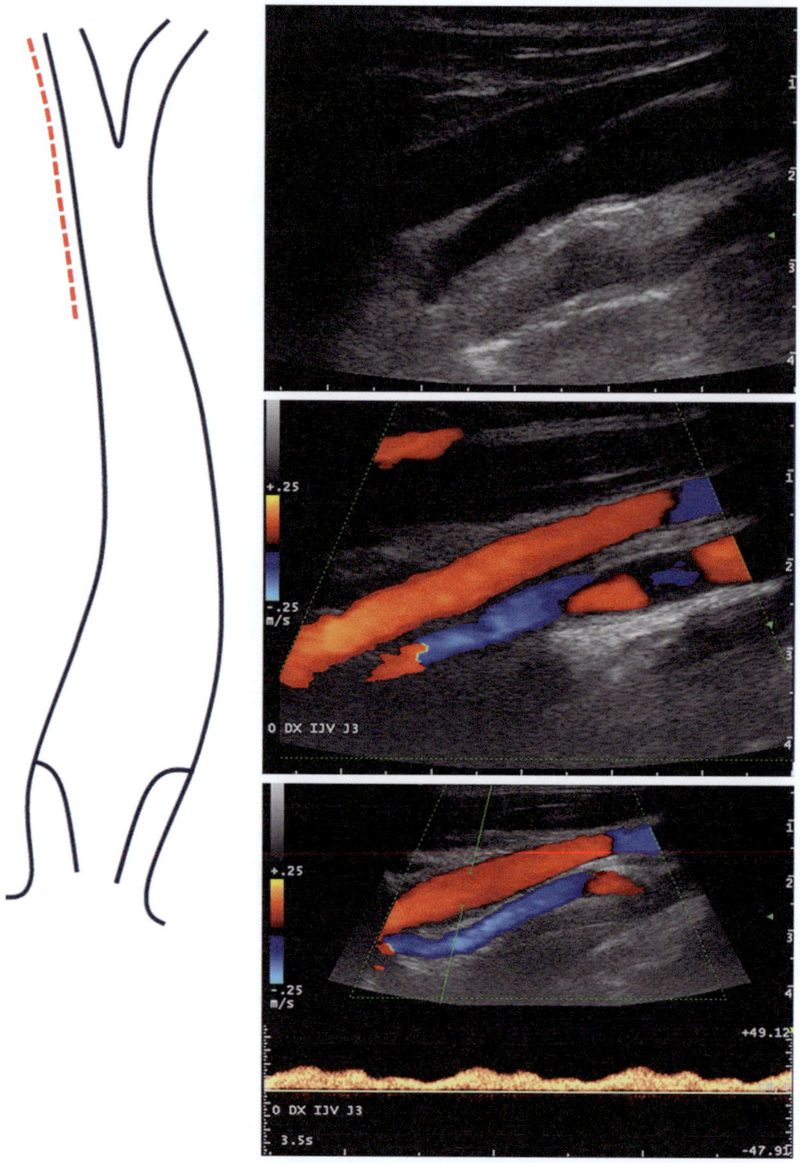

Fig. 2.13 Longitudinal scan of IJV at the level of the distal segment (J3). From *up* to *bottom*: (1) B-mode scan with J3 IJV (*yellow asterisk*) and carotid axis (*white asterisk*). (2) Image in color mode of the same structures, with the identification of the opposite direction between arteries and veins in the Doppler waveform (see also Movie 2.9). (3) J3 IJV Doppler waveform

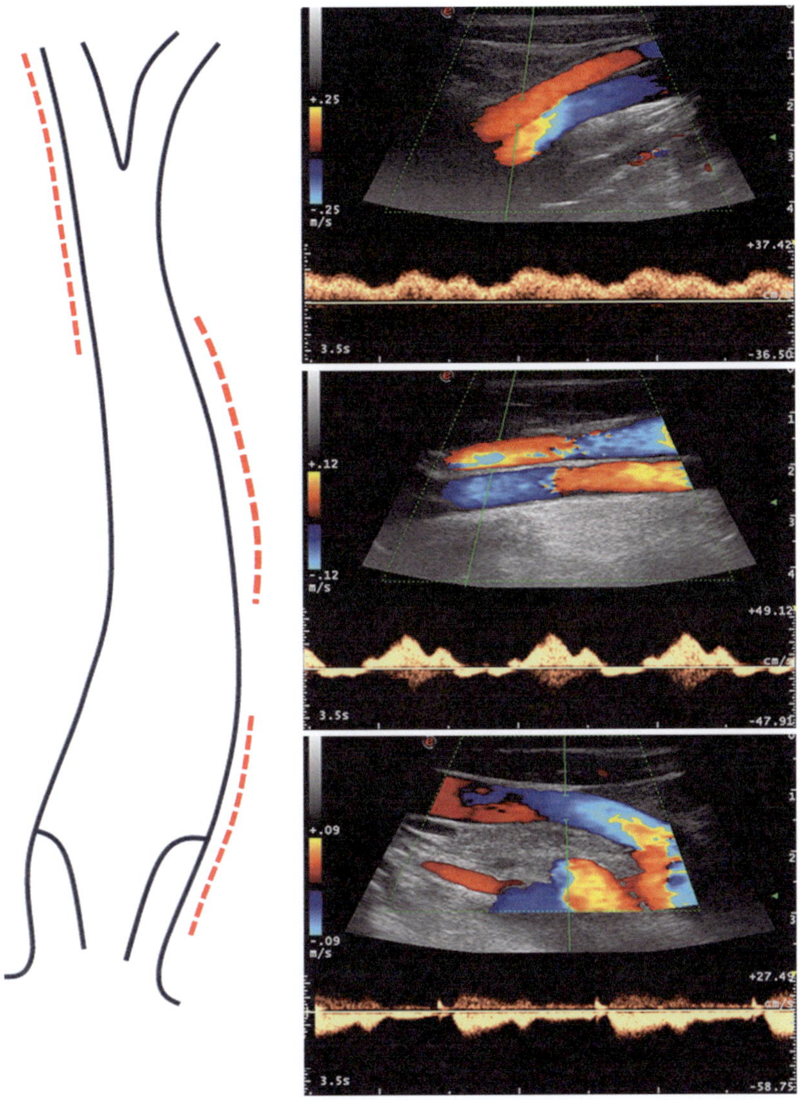

Fig. 2.14 Longitudinal scan of IJV at the level of J1, J2, and J3 in color mode and Doppler mode. From *top* to *bottom*, J1, J2, and J3 IJV are imaged; the variation of the Doppler waveform is showed, being similar to the one of central veins in J1–J2 segments, nearer to the *right* atrium, and partially different in the J3 segment, more distant from the *right* atrium

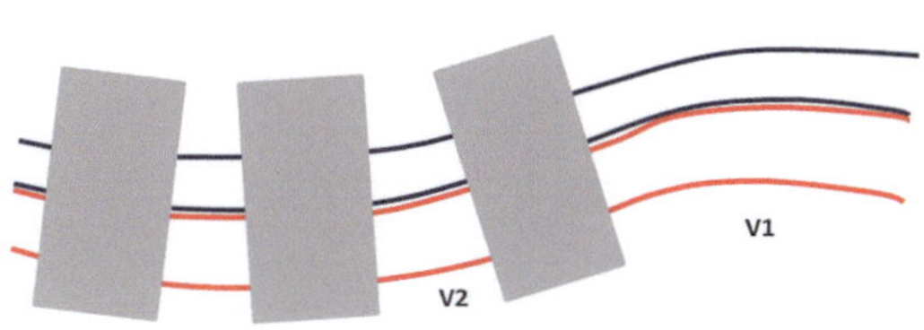

Fig. 2.15 Schematic drawing of the venous plexus of the VA at the V1 and V2 levels; VV is outlined in blue, and the vertebral artery is outlined in *red*; the *gray* boxes correspond to the shadows of the vertebral bones in the ultrasound image

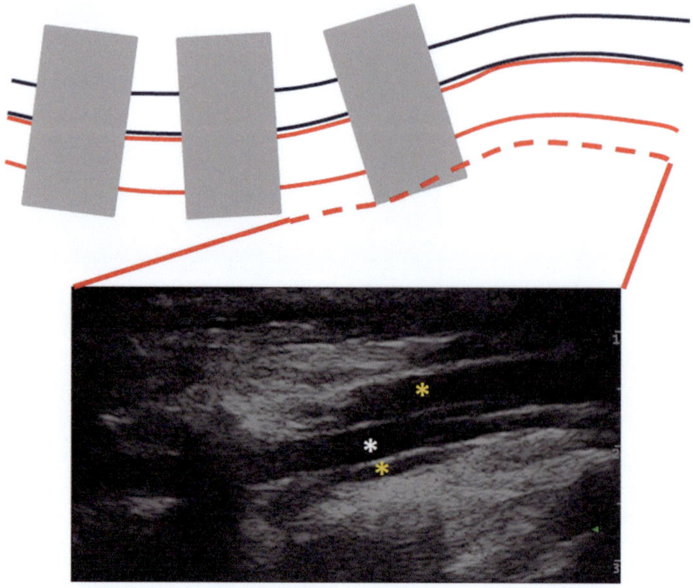

Fig. 2.16 Venous plexus of the vertebral artery at the level of V1 and proximal V2 segments in B-mode. The vertebral artery is indicated by the *white asterisk* and the venous plexus surrounding it by the *yellow asterisk*. The Movie 2.10 shows the dynamic relation between these structures

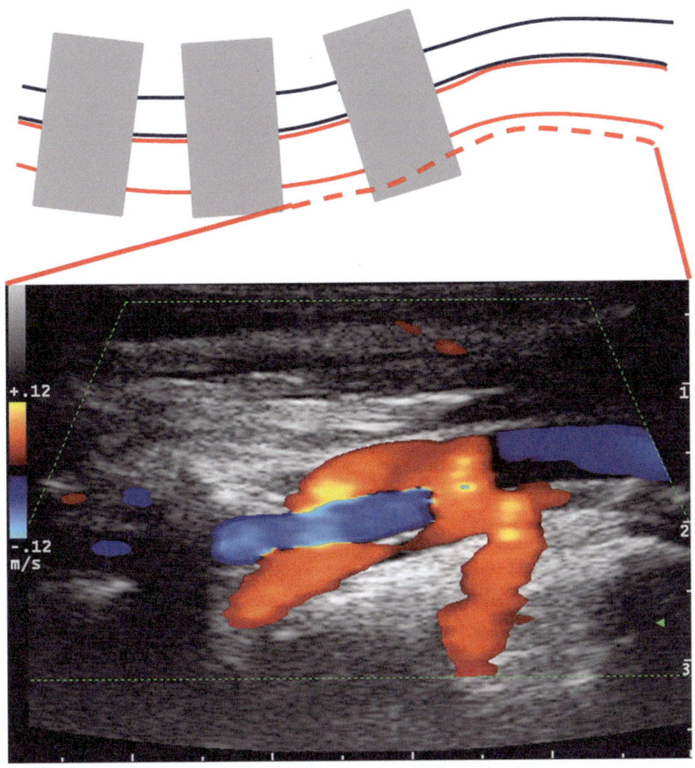

Fig. 2.17 VA venous plexus at the level of V1 and proximal V2 segments in color mode. The opposite color-coded signal of artery and vein corresponds to the different flow direction. It is evident the plexiform aspect of the vertebral venous outflow, surrounding the VA, and the confluence of at least one deep cervical branch (*green asterisk*), frequently found at this level, where the main trunk of the VV collects the flow from plexi and deep cervical veins before to join the SV. See Movie 2.11 about the relation between arteries and veins

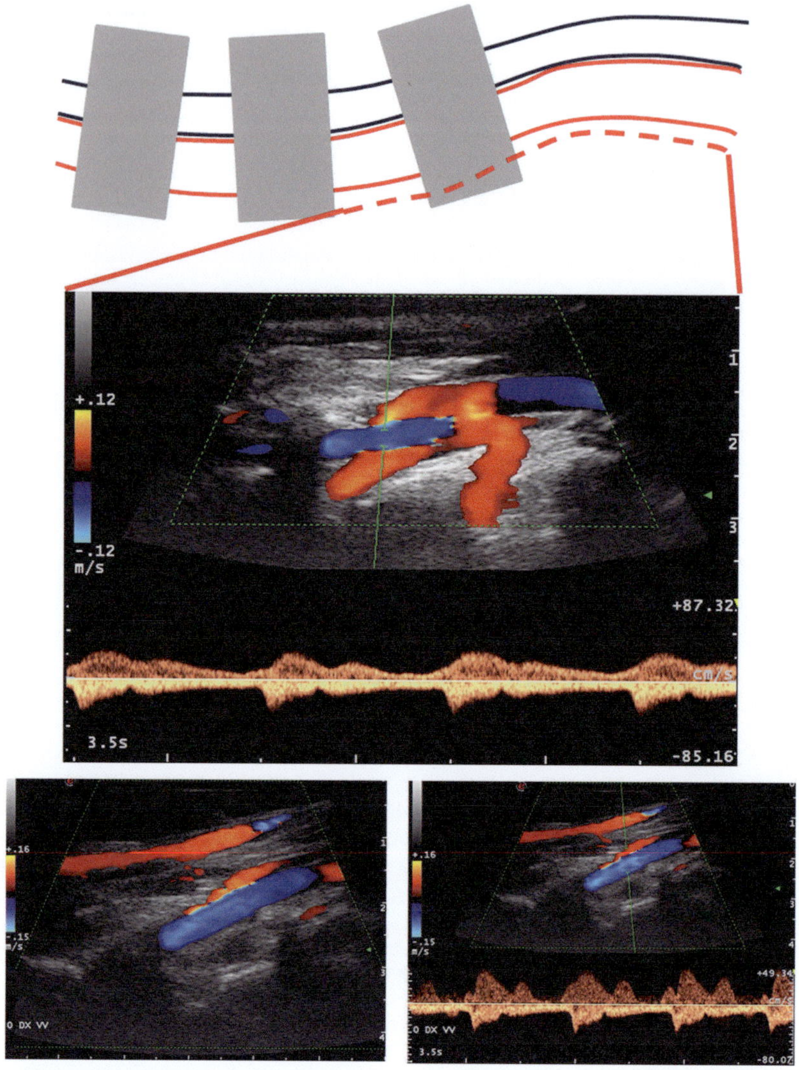

Fig. 2.18 Venous plexus of the VA at the level of V1 and proximal V2 segments in color mode and Doppler mode. In the examples, two features are represented: (1) the morphological variability of the plexus with more (*top* image) or less (*bottom* image) evident venous network and deep cervical veins confluence. (2) The Doppler waveform variability, more (*bottom* image) or less (*top* image) similar to the one of central veins

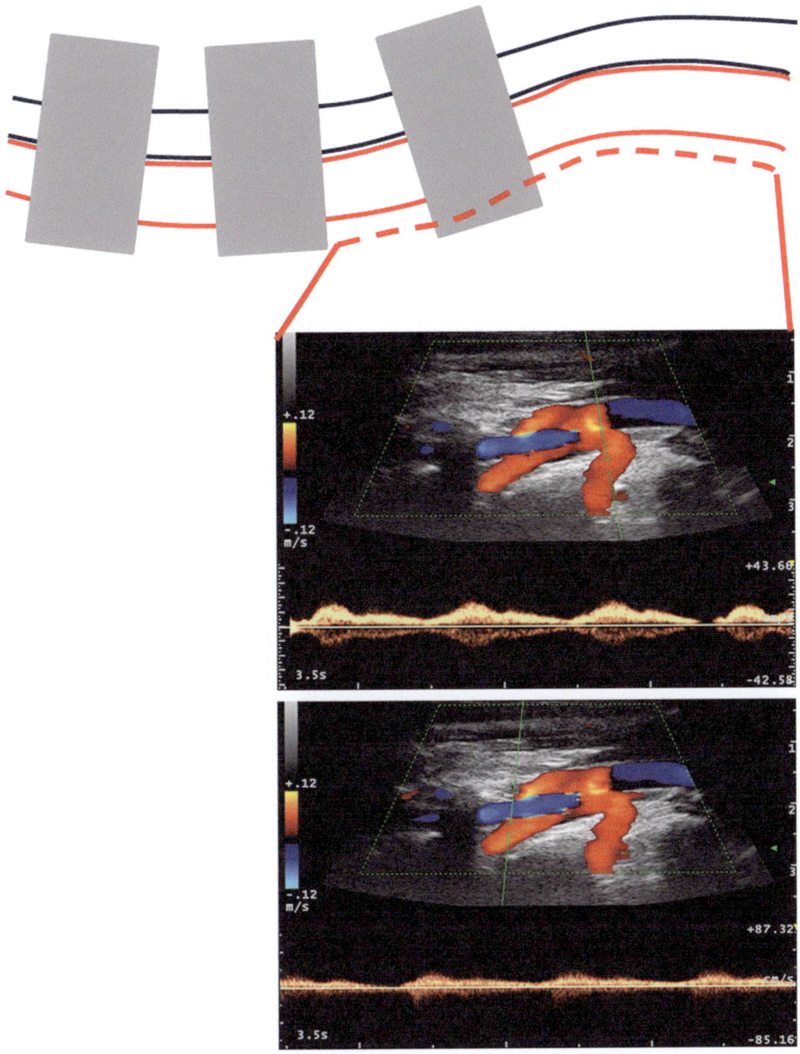

Fig. 2.19 VA venous plexus at the V1 and proximal V2 levels in color mode and Doppler mode. The entrance point of two deep cervical veins is identified and the Doppler waveform sampled, showing the same variability as IJV one depending on heart and breath cycles

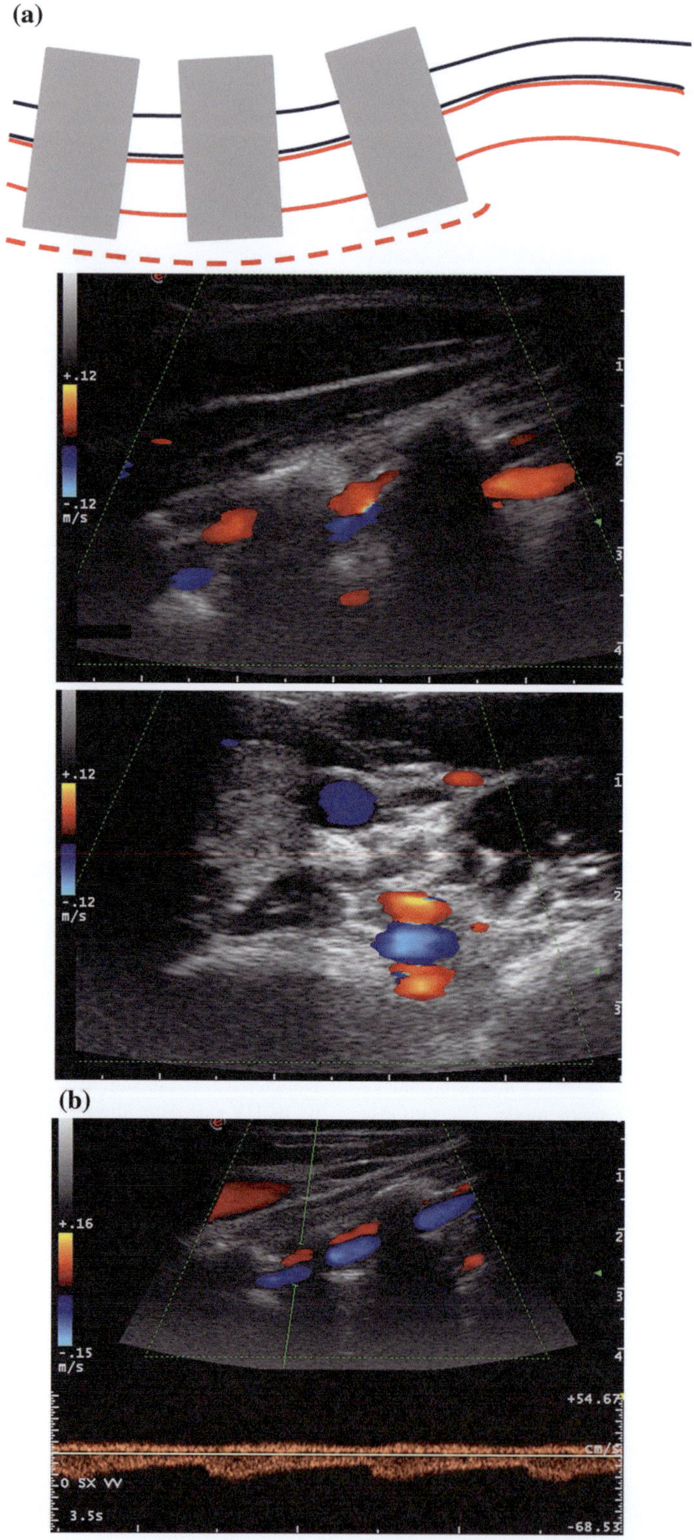

Fig. 2.20 VA venous plexus at the V2 level in color mode. **a** Longitudinal scan (*top image*) of the intertransverse channel along three sequential segments, where the VA and VV are recognizable, and transverse scan (*bottom image*) (see also Movie 2.12), confirming the network organization of the vertebral venous outflow (see also Movie 2.13). **b** VA and VV Doppler waveform at the V2 level

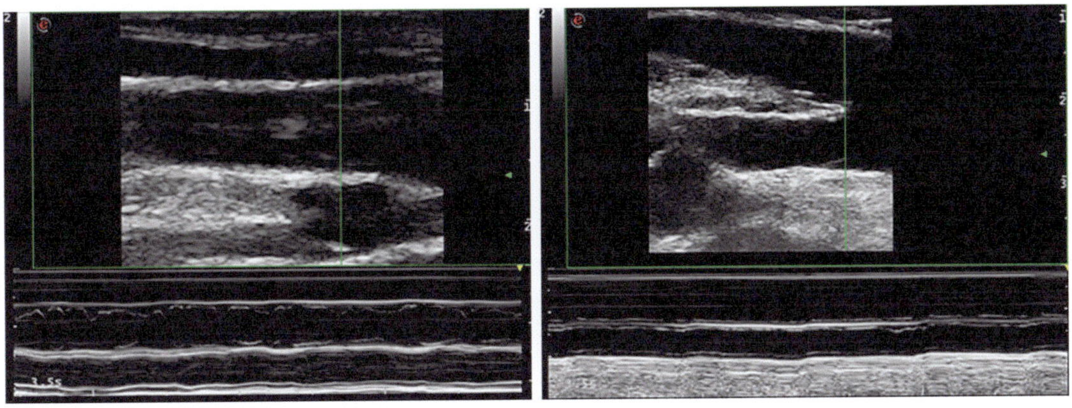

Fig. 2.21 VV valve in B-mode. As the IJV, also the VV has a valve system at the confluence into the SV and M-mode is as much suitable for its study

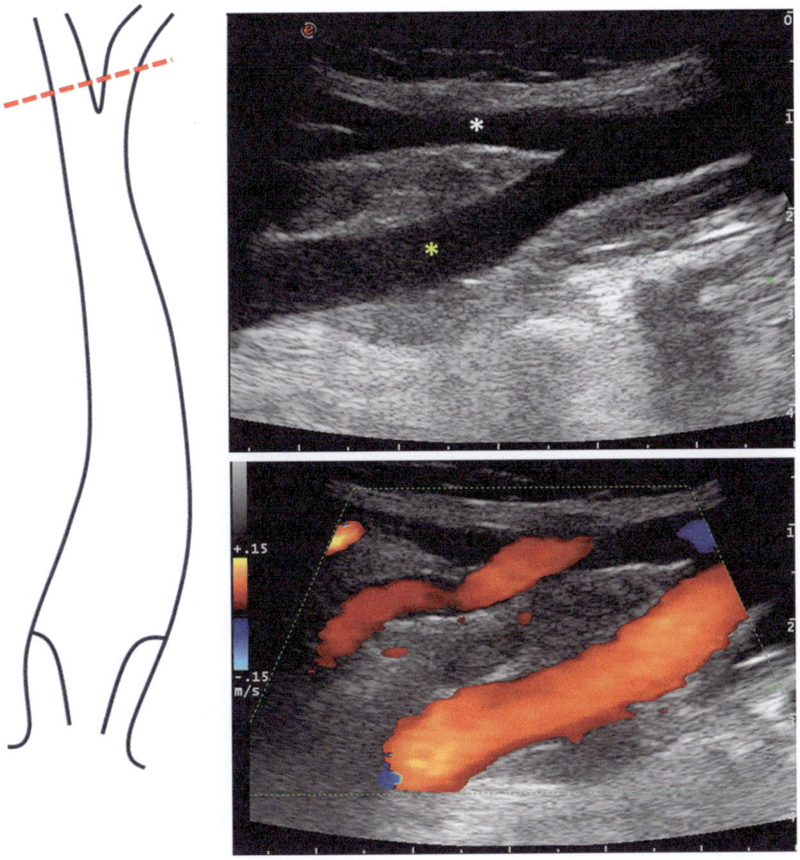

Fig. 2.22 IJV branches in longitudinal scan in B-mode and color mode. At the *top*, there is an image in B-mode with the lingual-facial trunk (*white asterisk*) and J3 IJV (*yellow asterisk*). In the *bottom* image, there is the correspondent structures in color mode (see also Movie 2.14)

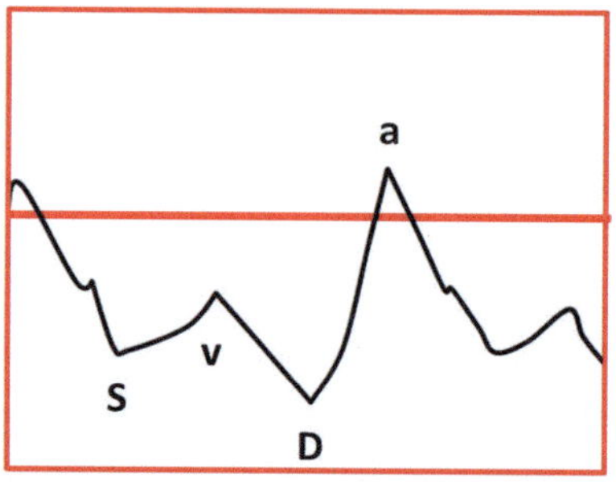

Fig. 2.23 Schematic drawing of the venous flow pattern in the *central* veins

References

1. Caruso RD, Rosenbaum AE, Chang JK et al (1999) Craniocervical junction venous anatomy on enhanced MR images: the suboccipital cavernous sinus. AJNR Am J Neuroradiol 20:1127–1131
2. Valdueza JM, von Munster T, Hoffman O et al (2000) Postural dependency of the cerebral venous outflow. Lancet 355:200–201
3. San Millan Ruiz D, Gailloud P, Rufenacht DA et al (2002) The craniocervical venous system in relation to cerebral venous drainage. AJNR Am J Neuroradiol, 23:1500–1508
4. Schreiber SJ, Lurtzing F, Gotze R et al (2003) Extrajugular pathways of human cerebral venous blood drainage assessed by duplex ultrasound. J Appl Physiol 94:1802–1805
5. Doepp F, Schreiber SJ, von Munster T et al (2004) How does the blood leave the brain? a systematic ultrasound analysis of cerebral venous drainage patterns. Neuroradiology 46:565–570
6. Seoane E, Rhoton AL (1999) Compression of the internal jugular vein by the transverse process of the atlas as the cause of cerebellar hemorrhage after supratentorial craniotomy. Surg Neurol 51:500–505
7. Lim CL, Keshava SN, Lea M (2006) Anatomical variations of the internal jugular veins and their relationship to the carotid arteries: a CT evaluation. Australas Radiol 50:314–318
8. Asouhidou I, Natsis K, Asteri T et al (2008) Anatomical variation of left internal jugular vein: clinical significance for an anaesthesiologist. Eur J Anesthiol 25:314–318
9. Troianos CA, Kuwik RJ, Pasqual JR, Lim AJ, Odasso DP (1996) Internal jugular vein and carotid artery anatomic relation as determined by ultrasonography. Anesthesiology 85(1):43–48
10. Hong JY, Koo BN, Kim WO, Choi E, Kil HK (2010) Effect of head rotation on overlap and relative position of internal jugular vein to carotid artery in infants and children: a study of the anatomy using ultrasonography. J Crit Care, 25(2):360.e9–360.e13. Epub 2010 Feb 10
11. Dresser LP, McKinney WM (1987) Anatomic and pathophysiologic studies of the human internal jugular valve. Am J Surg 154:220–224
12. Prades JM, Timoshenko A, Dumoillard JM et al (2002) High duplication of the internal jugular veins: clinical incidence in the adult and surgical consequences, a report of three clinical cases. Surg Radiol Anat 24:129–132
13. Lepori D, Capasso P, Fournier D, Genton CY, Schnyder P (1999) High-resolution ultrasound evaluation of internal jugular venous valves. Eur Radiol 9:1222–1226
14. Macchi C, Catini C (1994) The valves of the internal jugular veins, a statistical investigation in 120 living subjects using ultrasonic tomography. Ital J Anat Embryol 99:123–127
15. Darge K, Brandis U, Zieger B et al (2001) Internal jugular venous valves in children: high-resolution US findings. Eur Radiol 11:655–658
16. Midy D, Le Huee JC, Dumont D et al (1988) Etude anatomique et histologique des valves des veines jugulaires internes. Bull Assoc Anat 72:21–29
17. Anderhuber F (1984) Venous valves in the large branches of superior vena cava. Acta Anat (Basel) 119:184–192
18. Murase M, Maeda M, Teranishi K et al (1993) Morphological and functional study of internal jugular vein valve. Jpn J Cardiovasc Surg 22:383–386
19. Browlow RL, McKinney WM (1985) Ultrasonic evaluation of jugular venous valve competence. J Ultrasound Med 4:169–172
20. Lin BS, Kong CW, Tarng DC, Huang TP, Tang GJ (1998) Anatomical variation of the internal jugular vein and its impact on temporary haemodialysis vascular access: an ultrasonographic survey in uremic patients. Nephrol Dial Transplant 13:134–138
21. Taal MW, Chesteron LJ, McIntyre CW (2004) Venography at insertion of tunneled internal jugular vein dialysis catheters reveals significant occult stenosis. Nephrol Dial Transplant 19:1542–1545
22. Lim CL, Keshava SN, Lea M (2006) Anatomical variations of the internal jugular veins and their relationship to the carotid arteries: a CT evaluation. Australas Radiol 50:314–318
23. Tartiere D, Seguin P, Jubel C, Laviolle B, Malledant Y (2009) Estimation of the diameter and cross-sectional area of the internal jugular veins in adult patients. Crit Care 13:R197
24. Mortensen JD, Talbot S, Burkart JA (1990) Cross-sectional internal diameters of human cervical and femoral blood vessels: relationship to subject's sex, age, and body size. Anat Rec 225:115–124
25. Escott EJ, Branstetter BF (2006) It's not a cervical lymph node, it's a vein: CT and MR imaging findings in the veins of the head and neck. Radiographics 26:1501–1515

26. Suarez T, Baerwald JP, Kraus C (2002) Central venous access: the effects of approach, position, and head rotation on internal jugular vein crosssectional area. Anesth Analg 95:1519–1524
27. Muhammad JK, Pugh ND, Boden L, Crean SJ, Fardy MJ (2001) The effect of head rotation on the diameter of the internal jugular vein: implications for free tissue transfer. J Craniomaxillofac Surg 29:214–218
28. Paleri V, Gopalakrishnan S (2001) Jugular phlebectasia: theory of pathogenesis and review of literature. Int J Pediatr Otorhinolaryngol 57:155–159
29. Chao HC, Wong KS, Lin SJ, Kong MS, Lin TY (1999) Ultrasonographic diagnosis and color flow Doppler sonography of internal jugular venous ectasia in children. J Ultrasound Med 18:411–416
30. Shima H, von Luedinghausen M, Ohno K et al (1998) Anatomy of microvascular anastomosis in the neck. Plast Reconstr Surg 101:33–41
31. Silva MA, Deen KI, Fernando DJS et al (2002) The internal jugular vein valve may have a significant role in the prevention of venous reflux: evidence from live and cadaveric human subjects. Clin Physiol Funct Imaging 22:202–205
32. Chung CP, Hsu HY, Chao AC et al (2007) Flow volume in the jugular vein and related hemodynamics in the branches of the jugular vein. Ultrasound Med Biol 33:500–505
33. Comert E, Comert A (2009) External jugular vein duplication. J Craniofac Surg 20:2173–2174
34. Williams PL, Warwick R, Dyson M, Bannister LH (eds) (1989) Gray's anatomy, 37th edn. Edinburgh, Churchill-Livingstone
35. Deslaugiers B, Vaysse P, Combes JM et al (1994) Contribution to the study of the tributaries and the termination of the external jugular vein. Surg Radiol Anat 16:173–177
36. Schummer W, Schummer C, Bredle D, Frober R (2004) The anterior jugular venous system: variability and clinical impact. Anesth Analg 99:1625–1629
37. Andeweg J (1996) The anatomy of collateral venous flow from the brain and its value in aetiological interpretation of intracranial pathology. Neuroradiology 38:621–689
38. Epstein HM, Linde HW, Crampton AR et al (1970) The vertebral venous plexus as a major cerebral venous outflow tract. Anesthesiology 32:332–337
39. Batson OV (1957) The vertebral vein system. AJR Am J Roentgenol 78:195–212
40. Cooper ERA (1960) The vertebral venous plexus. Acta Anat 42:333–351
41. Caruso RD, Rosenbaum AE, Chang JK et al (1999) Craniocervical junction venous anatomy on enhanced MR images: the suboccipital cavernous sinus. AJNR Am J Neuroradiol 20:1127–3119
42. Osborn AG (1980) Introduction to cerebral angiography. Harper & Row, New York
43. Cummings CW (1935) Otolaryngology: head and neck surgery. Mosby Books, Philadelphia

3 Postural Changes and Activation Tests

3.1 Postural Changes

The cerebral venous outflow depends mainly on body position, as demonstrated also by using a mathematical model by Gisolf [1]. Indeed in supine position, IJVs of most people are the main drainage routes for cerebral venous flow both about the blood volume and about the blood flow, whereas in upright position, IJV has a negative intraluminal pressure, being located above the heart level, and therefore, it is more easily collapsible [2]. In upright position, the vertebral venous plexus represents an alternative drainage route, whose activation is position dependent, being usually less efficient in supine position [3]. The positive pressure breath demonstrated to be able to reopen IJV in upright position both in dogs [4] and in men [2]. With the aim of studying the responses of jugular and vertebral venous system to the changes of body position, Gisolf and colleagues [1] proposed a mathematical model showing the different blood flow distribution between the jugular and vertebral axis in supine and upright position, considering the vertebral axis/plexus as alternative route, also including the effects of the Valsalva maneuver. They applied this mathematical model on healthy volunteers in comparison with ultrasound techniques. Depending on the physiological data from which the model was derived, IJV is the main route of drainage in supine position and probably it collapses in upright position, so decreasing its blood flow. An increase in the intracerebral pressure until 40 mmHg should be sufficient to transiently reopen IJV.

The results derived from the application of the model were confirmed by ultrasound imaging concerning CSA of IJV in supine and upright position, adding the Valsalva maneuver. In upright position, the IJV collapse causes an increase in the resistance to cerebral venous outflow, and other routes open, as the vertebral venous plexus. Performing a Valsalva maneuver in upright position further increases the cerebral venous pressure, decreasing the resistance to the outflow and reopening IJVs. All daily activities associated with the phase II b of the Valsalva maneuver (straining phase) determine the same effect on the cerebral venous outflow. In the computer simulation during the straining phase of Valsalva maneuver in upright position, also a decrease in the blood flow of the vertebral venous plexus occurs. However, previous studies of Batson demonstrated that, during the straining phase, the flow direction in the vertebral venous plexus changes, becoming caudocranial [5, 6].

Electronic supplementary material Supplementary material is available in the online version of this chapter at http://dx.doi.org/10.1007/978-88-470-5465-3_3. Videos can also be accessed at http://www.springerimages.com/videos/978-88-470-5465-3

G. Malferrari et al., *Neurosonological Evaluation of Cerebral Venous Outflow*,
DOI: 10.1007/978-88-470-5465-3_3, © Springer-Verlag Italia 2014

The main limitation of this simplified model concerns the need of a more precise characterization of the vertebral venous plexus from the physical point of view for two reasons: The first one is the presence of the multiple anastomoses, better described by the association of a resistor and a capacitor (this last one is affected by the central venous pressure), and the second one is the presence of extrajugular and extravertebral outflow routes (e.g., deep cervical veins), able to be differently activated and efficient either in supine and in upright position in normal subjects [7, 8]. Another cause of variability that makes difficult to widely apply this model in individual cases is the frequent asymmetry of IJV in size and function among the two sides. This asymmetry in size often causes significant side-by-side difference in the IJV venous outflow. Moreover, the IJV collapse occurs already by 30–35° tilting [9], and a significant decrease in the IJV outflow occurs can be seen already at 15° tilting angle [10]. Again a mildest tilting (10°) in the opposite direction, i.e., with the head down starting from a supine position, causes an increase in IJV CSA [11].

Further information about the physiology of the cerebral venous outflow in supine and upright (or seated) position came from neuroradiological studies using magnetic resonance imaging (MRI) techniques on healthy volunteers [12]. Despite the few subjects, the finding of this last study has a relevance to define the physiological variability of the normal people: Indeed, about a half of the cerebral venous outflow by IJV, going from the supine to the seated position, shifts on secondary venous channels (vertebral, epidural, and deep cervical veins) without a significant reduction in the global outflow (a decrease of only 12 % in seated position was documented), contrary to what previously reported by Valdueza and colleagues 10], about the 75 % decrease in global venous outflow, and the 90 % decrease in the IJV outflow in seated position. This difference, coming from two studies with a small sample of subjects, could be inferred to be due to the wide inter-individual variability in the venous drainage as well as to the difference between ultrasound and MRI techniques.

Another relevant item raised from this study is that the dynamic balance between venous outflow and arterial inflow is also dependent on the biomechanic status of the cerebrovascular system. Indeed in seated position, a significant reduction in the venous outflow pulsatility is found without changes in the pulsatility of the arterial inflow. This point could be explained by the increased compliance of the venous routes system (2.8-fold increase in the intracranial compliance index), i.e., by a decreased blood volume in this vessels in upright position in comparison with the supine position, according to the gravity [13].

3.2 Activation Tests

Either ultrasound or MRI studies on healthy volunteers using the phase contrast technique at the IJV level [14] confirmed the physiological data about the relation between the breath cycle and IJV flow parameters, both for size and for the measure of the blood flow.

During the inspiration, the intrathoracic pressure decreases, becoming more negative and reducing the resistance to outflow for the IJV, while during the expiration, the intrathoracic pressure increases, becoming less negative and increasing the resistance to the IJV outflow. Therefore, lacking diseases that can affect the central venous pressure and significant valve incontinence, it should be expected that IJV CSA progressively decreases during inspiration and increases during expiration. Moreover, confirming this relation between IJV CSA and the breath cycle, the application of an end-expiratory positive pressure can increase IJV CSA until a maximal value correspondent to a positive pressure of 12 cm H_2O [15].

The more known and standardized activation test is the Valsalva maneuver, whose effects on the central venous pressure are well studied and demonstrated. The Valsalva maneuver defines a forced expiration against a closed glottis; during each phase, different changes occur in several parameters, as intrathoracic pressure, and consequently in venous outflow, cardiac output, arterial pressure, heart rate, and so on. The starting phase of a Valsalva maneuver involves the contraction of diaphragm and intercostal muscles, that make the intrathoracic pressure positive, though a compression of the thoracic great vessels and cardiac chambers. The association of venous compression and increased right atrial pressure increases the resistance to the cerebral venous outflow into the central veins. The transiently decreased cardiac filling causes a cardiac output reduction, but it is associated with a transient increase in aortic pressure because of the compression of the thoracic aorta causes (phase I).

In phase II, the aortic pressure progressively falls, following the fall in cardiac output, and the heart rate increases.

At the release of Valsalva maneuver, starting the normal breath, the aortic pressure briefly decreases, and consequently, heart rate briefly increases (phase III).

In the phase IV, the cardiac filling increases and causes an increase in aortic pressure.

The phase II or straining is the most interesting phase about venous return, because there is a reduction in venous drainage because of the increased intrathoracic pressure.

The role of the phase II (particularly IIb or straining phase) as activation test for the study of venous hemodynamics is detailed in the next chapter with the standardization of the application of this maneuver.

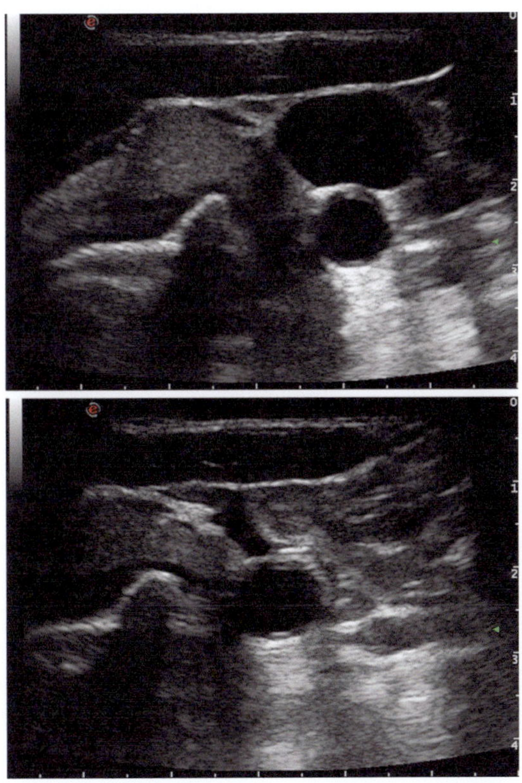

Fig. 3.1 J2 IJV segment in transverse scanning plane. Sometimes there is a huge variation between IJV expiratory CSA (*figure above*) and inspiratory CSA (*figure below*) during normal breath. See the corresponding movie of breath dynamics (Movie 3.1)

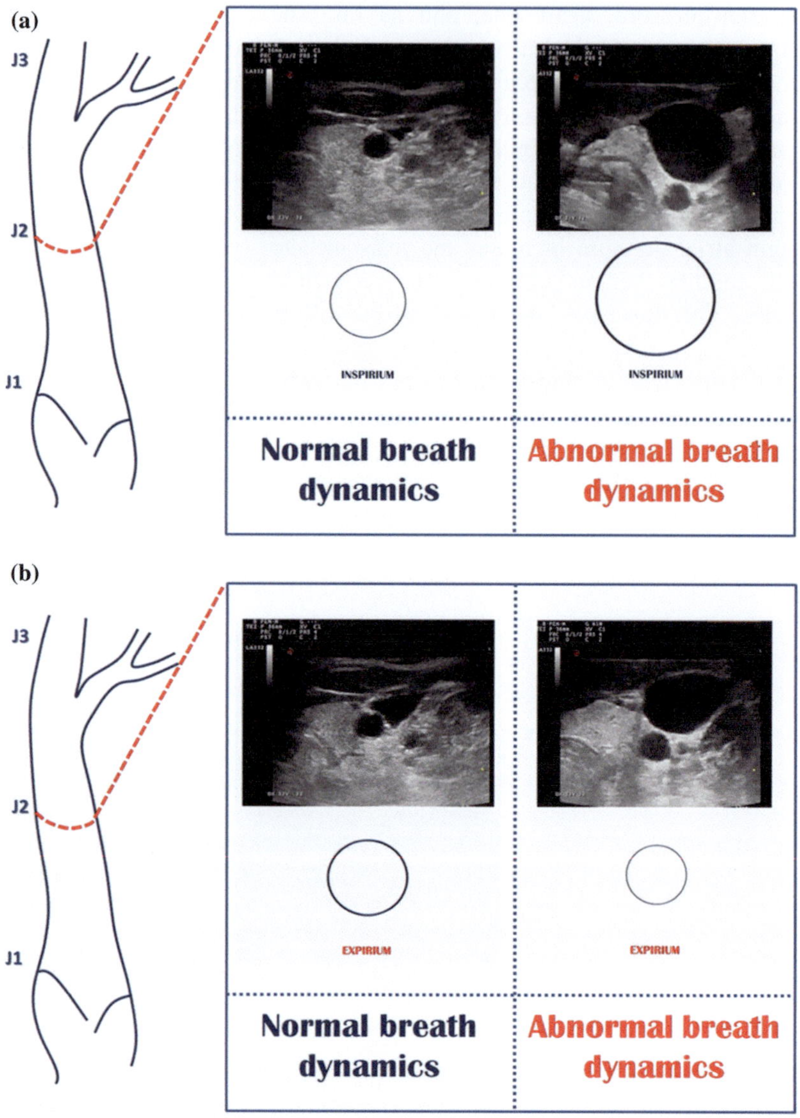

Fig. 3.2 Schematic drawing of J2 IJV CSA variations during normal breath in a normal subject (i.e., a subject whose responses are congruent with the physiological data described in the chapter) (*left* side of the image) and in a subject with opposite behavior (*right* side of the image), during inspiration (Fig. 3.2a) and in the end-expiratory phase (Fig. 3.2b). See also Movie 3.2

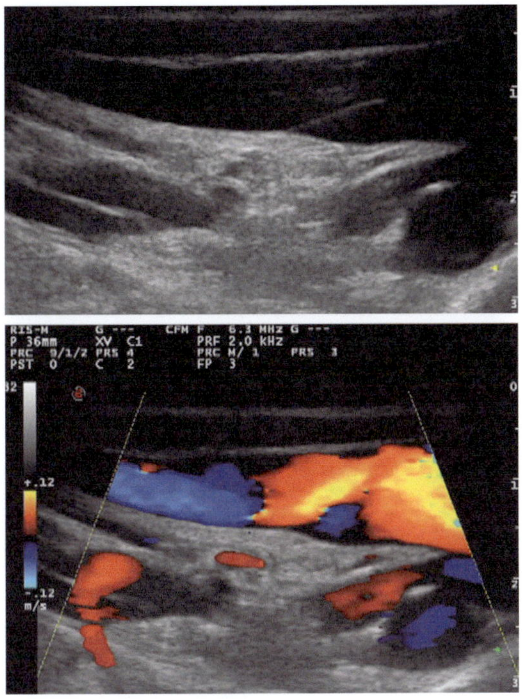

Fig. 3.3 Longitudinal scan of J1 IJV in B-mode and in color mode during normal breath. In B-mode (*top picture*), the two valve leaflets opening can be seen. In color mode (*bottom picture*), an orthodromic flow of IJV is evident with the posterior leaflet separating the orthodromic flow laminae from the valve sinus, where a minimal stasis with retrograde filling is normal

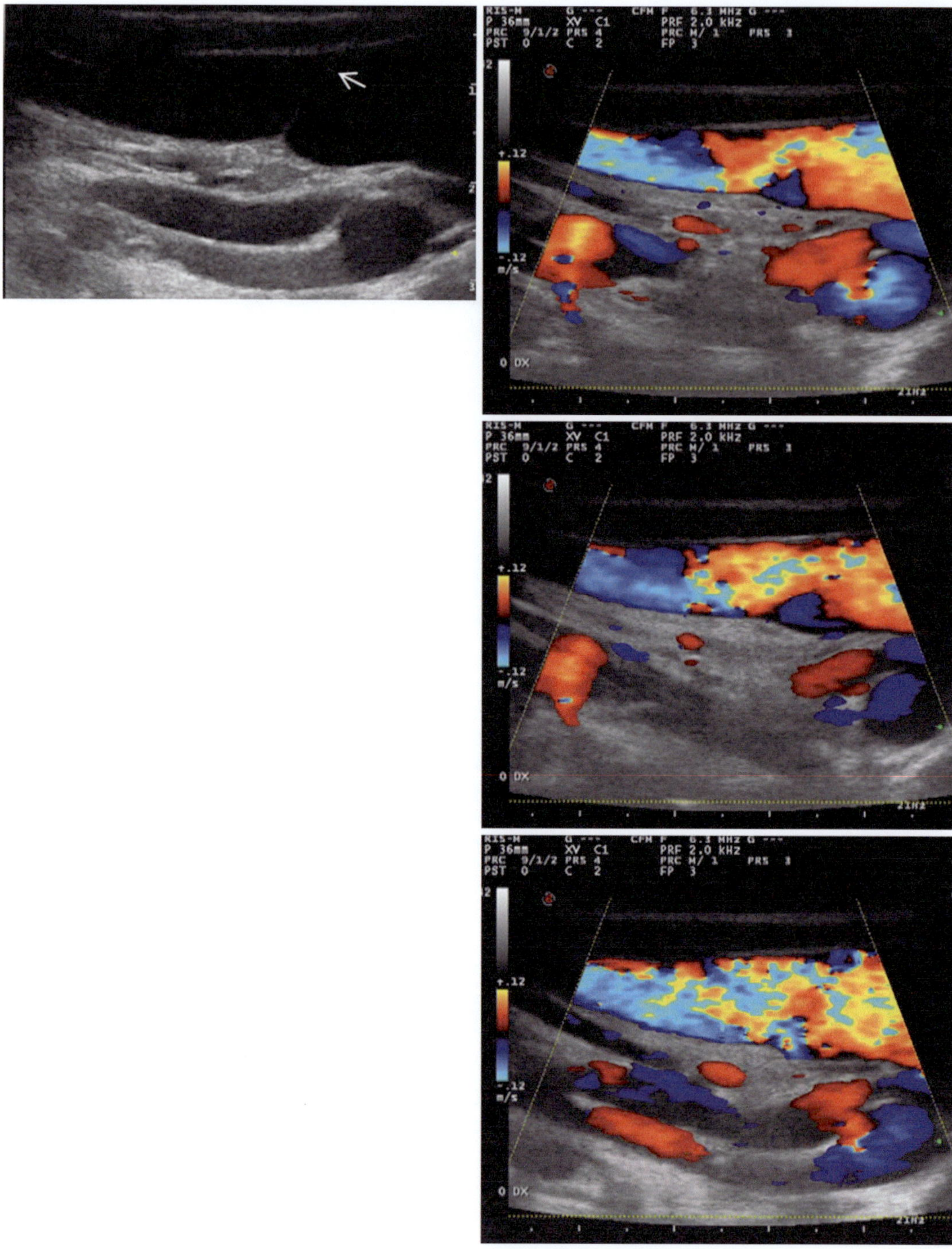

Fig. 3.4 Longitudinal scan of J1 IJV in B-mode and in color mode during the Valsalva maneuver. In B-mode (*top left picture*), it is well evident the quite perfect closeness of the valve leaflets with a minimal discontinuity (*arrow*) (see also Movie 3.3). In color mode, the three sequential images show from *top* to *bottom right picture* that the regurgitation jet progressively fills the prevalvular IJV segment with an increasing aliasing, as in the Movie 3.4

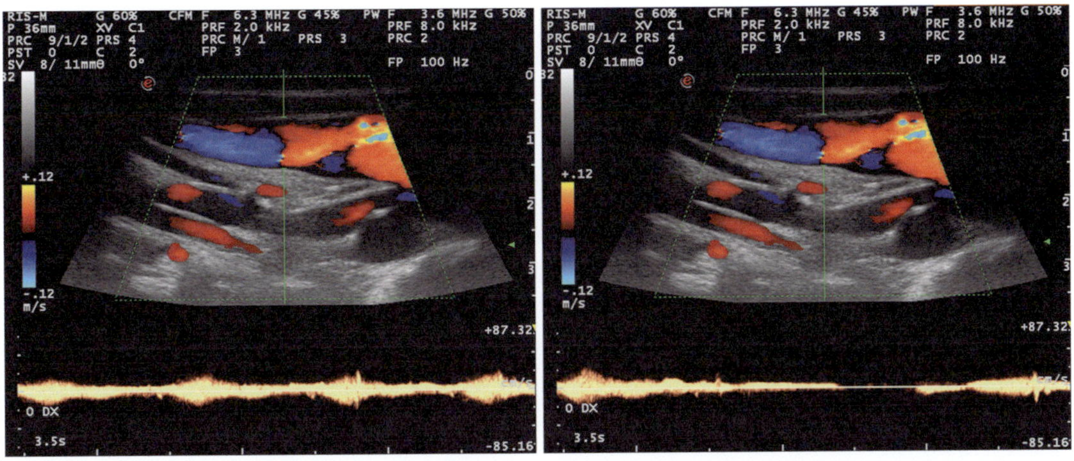

Fig. 3.5 Longitudinal scan of J1 IJV in color mode. In the *above picture*, the Doppler waveform is sampled during normal breath, near the valve plan, without evident reflux. In the *picture below*, the Doppler waveform is sampled during the straining phase of the Valsalva maneuver, eliciting a flow decrease near to zero

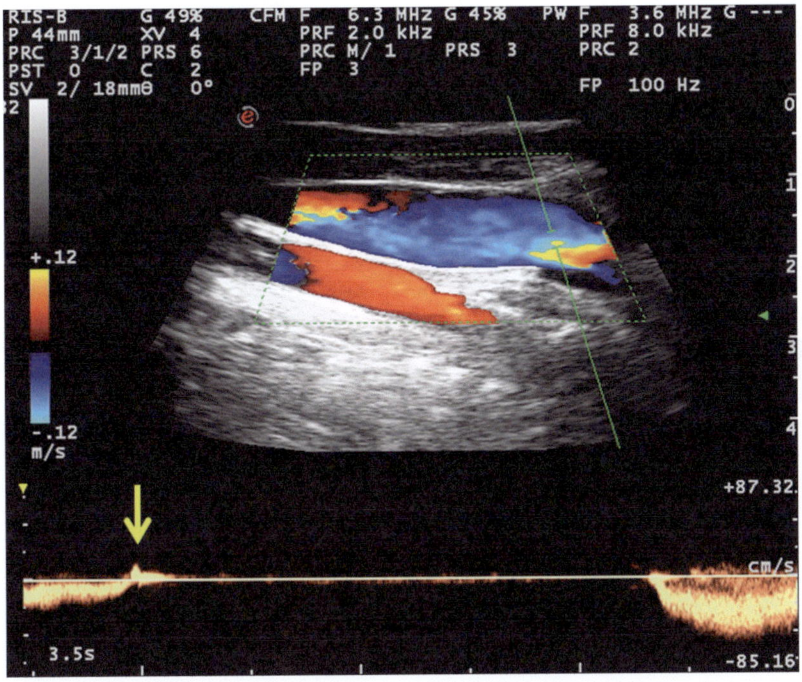

Fig. 3.6 IJV valve continence with Valsalva maneuver. The sample volume is slightly above the valve plan in the lumen of the IJV in Duplex mode. The waveform below has been acquired with Valsalva maneuver, and it shows an abrupt stop of the venous flow after a very short physiological flow reversal (*yellow arrow*). The corresponding stop of blood flow in color mode is illustrated in the Movie 3.5

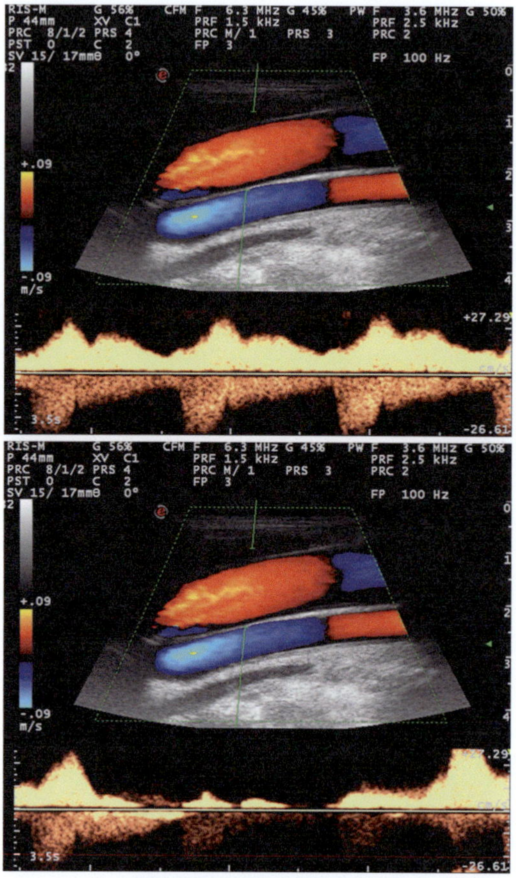

Fig. 3.7 Longitudinal scan of J2 IJV in color mode. In the *above picture*, there is a normal variation of the Doppler waveform with the breath cycle. The flow direction of IJV is opposite in comparison with the one of the accompanying CCA (see also Movie 3.6). In the *picture below*, the same IJV segment is studied, applying the Valsalva maneuver. In the Doppler waveform, it can be seen the initial inversion of flow direction (*yellow arrow*) and the subsequent orthograde rebound with very low velocity during the straining phase with increased flow at the release of straining (see Movie 3.7)

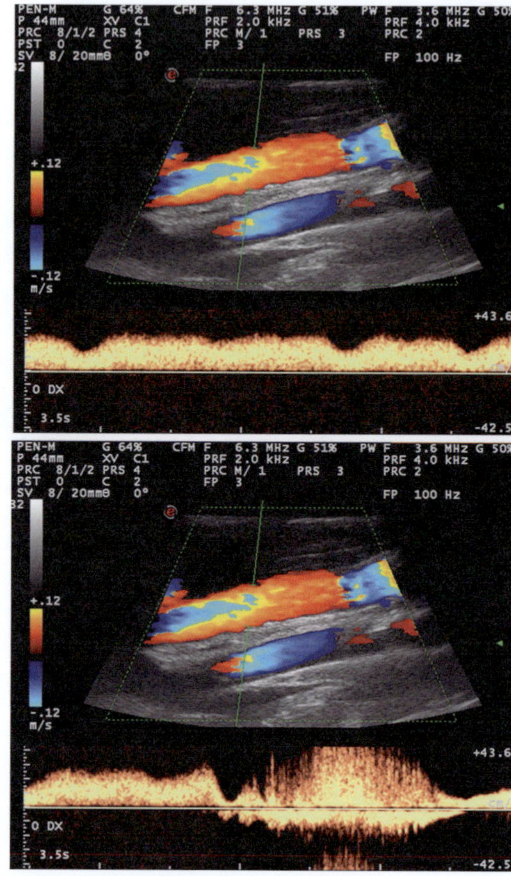

Fig. 3.8 Longitudinal scan of J2 IJV in color mode. In the *above picture*, there is a normal breath variation of the Doppler waveform with opposite direction in comparison with the CCA. In the *picture below*, during Valsalva maneuver, it can be seen a turbulent bidirectional flow component, as in the Movie 3.8

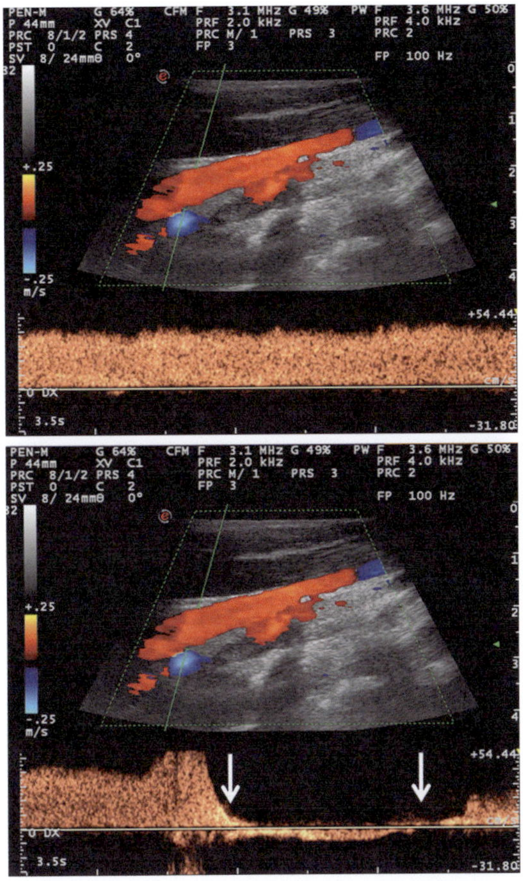

Fig. 3.9 Longitudinal scan of J3 IJV in color mode. In the above picture, there is a normal variation of the Doppler waveform with the breath, in opposite flow direction in comparison with the ICA. In the *picture below*, during Valsalva maneuver, it can be seen the inversion of flow direction (limited by the *two arrows*), as in the Movie 3.9

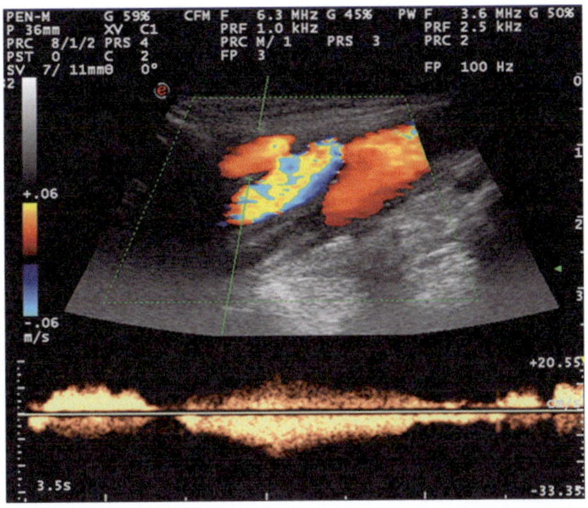

Fig. 3.10 Longitudinal scan of J3 IJV in color mode. There is another example of J3 IJV truncular incontinence during the Valsalva maneuver

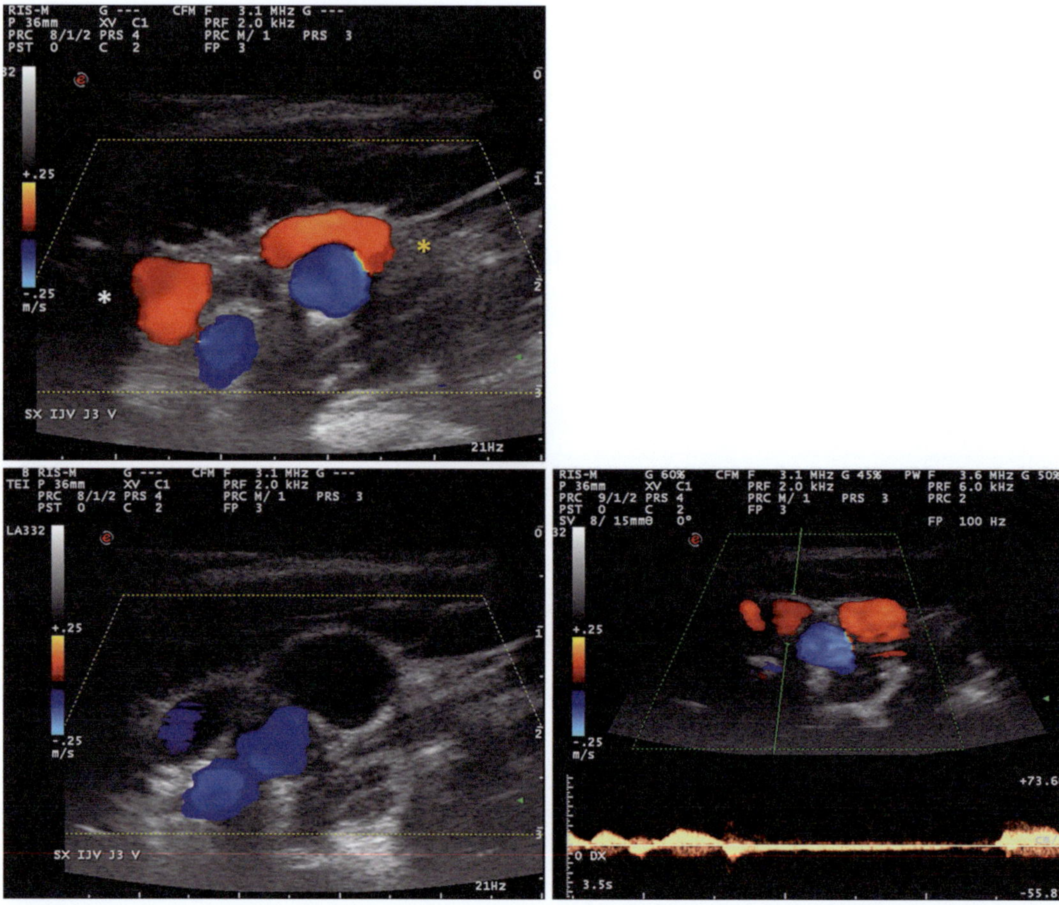

Fig. 3.11 Transverse scan of J3 IJV in color mode. In the *above picture*, it can be seen during normal breath the common facial vein (*white asterisk*) with an orthograde flow direction in comparison with J3 IJV (*yellow asterisk*). In the *picture below*, the application of Valsalva maneuver elicits the inversion of flow direction of the common facial vein and the decrease in flow to zero on the J3 IJV. In the correspondent Doppler waveform (below to the *right*), there is further confirmation of the inverted flow direction of the J3 IJV branch (see also Movie 3.10)

References

1. Gisolf J, van Lieshout JJ, van Heusden K, Pott F, Stok WJ, Karemaker JM (2004) Human cerebral venous outflow pathway depends on posture and central venous pressure. J Physiol 560:317–327
2. Cirovic S, Walsh C, Fraser WD, Gulino A (2003) The effect of posture and positive pressure breathing on the hemodynamics of the internal jugular vein. Aviat Space Environ Med 74:125–131
3. Chaynes P, Verdie JC, Moscovici J, Zadeh J, Vaysse P, Becue J (1998) Microsurgical anatomy of the internal vertebral venous plexuses. Surg Radiol Anat 20:47–51
4. Toung TJK, Aizawa H, Traystman RJ (2000) Effects of positive end-expiratory pressure ventilation on cerebral venous pressure with head elevation in dogs. J Appl Physiol 88:655–661
5. Batson OV (1957) The vertebral vein system. AJR Am J Roentgenol 78:195–212
6. Cooper ERA (1960) The vertebral venous plexus. Acta Anat 42:333–351
7. Schreiber SJ, Lurtzing F, Gotze R et al (2003) Extrajugular pathways of human cerebral venous blood drainage assessed by duplex ultrasound. J Appl Physiol 94:1802–1805
8. Doepp F, Schreiber SJ, von Munster T et al (2004) How does the blood leave the brain? A systematic ultrasound analysis of cerebral venous drainage patterns. Neuroradiology 46:565–570

9. Dawson EA, Secher NH, Dalsgaard MK, Ogoh S, Yoshiga CC, Gonzalez-Alonso J, Steensberg A, Raven PB (2004) Standing up to the challenge of standing: a siphon does not support cerebral blood flow in humans. Am J Physiol Regul Integr Comp Physiol 287:R911–R914
10. Valdueza JM, von Munster T, Hoffman O et al (2000) Postural dependency of the cerebral venous outflow. Lancet 355:200–201
11. Schreiber SJ, Lambert UK, Doepp F, Valdueza JM (2002) Effects of prolonged head down tilt on internal jugular vein cross-sectional area. Br J Anaesth 89:769–771
12. Alperin N, Lee SH, Sivaramakrishnan A, Hushek SG (2005) Quantifying the effect of posture on intracranial physiology in humans by MRI flow studies. J Magn Reson Imaging 22:591–596
13. Alperin N, Lee SH, Mazda M, Hushek SG, Roitberg B, Goddwin J, Lichtor T (2005) Evidence for the importance of extracranial venous flow in patients with idiopathic intracranial hypertension (IIH). Acta Neurochir Suppl 95:129–132
14. Schrauben et al (2012) Respiratory effects on phase contrast imaging of the jugular vein. J Cardiovasc Magnetic Resonance 14(Suppl 1):W4
15. LEE SC, HAN SS, SHIN SY, LIM YJ, KIM JT, KIM YH (2012) Relationship between positive end-expiratory pressure and internal jugular vein cross-sectional area, Acta Anesthesiologica Scandinavica Acta Anaesthesiol Scand, 56(7):840–845

4 Main Pathological Pictures with Ultrasound

4.1 Internal Jugular Vein Valves and Incontinence

The jugular vein valve system is located near the confluence of the IJV into the BCV. Its function is to prevent the retrograde flow toward the brain in case of sudden increase in intrathoracic pressure that may cause a transvalvular gradient up to 100 mmHg [1].

Besides, valve incontinence has been considered to be one of the possible causes in the onset of some neurological diseases (transient global amnesia, primary exertional headache, normotensive hydrocephalus). Also for this reason, the jugular valve continence is of crucial importance in ensuring the development of a transcranial pressure gradient during cardiopulmonary resuscitation with thoracic compression [2].

Coughing, vomiting, abdominal compression, yawning, hiccups, weeping as well as physical exertion are physiological conditions in which there may be a sudden increase in intrathoracic pressure and consequently a regurgitation into the IJV in case of valve incontinence. In some conditions, such a reflux has been proved to be able to reach the intracranial veins [3]. An association has been speculated between jugular valve incontinence and various neurological diseases which may be caused or sustained by a high intrathoracic pressure, such as transient global amnesia, frequently triggered by Valsalva-like activities [4–7]. Adding up the populations examined in these studies, jugular valve incontinence has been identified in 75.4 % of 114 patients affected by transient global amnesia, compared to 36.8 % of healthy control subjects.

Jugular valve incontinence is an incomplete leaflet closure, with blood reflux of variable volume and duration with a retrograde direction toward the brain starting from the valve plane. It is one of the most common pathological situations at the level of the cervical vein axis. Valve incontinence has been variously defined in the literature, with different criteria in each study. It has been evaluated both in normal breathing conditions and in situation of activation (Valsalva maneuver), until it has reached a methodological standardization with the identification of a duration threshold, with high and reproducible sensitivity and specificity. Among the different methods reported in the literature for the identification and evaluation of valve incontinence, the following are some of the most relevant ones:

- A semiquantitative grading has been adopted in the field of anesthesiology, i.e., in the evaluations on the jugular vein catheterization and on the guiding role of ultrasound methodology [8]. The grading ranges from 0 to 4, and it takes into account both the duration and

Electronic supplementary material Supplementary material is available in the online version of this chapter at http://dx.doi.org/10.1007/978-88-470-5465-3_4. Videos can also be accessed at http://www.springerimages.com/videos/978-88-470-5465-3

G. Malferrari et al., *Neurosonological Evaluation of Cerebral Venous Outflow*,
DOI: 10.1007/978-88-470-5465-3_4, © Springer-Verlag Italia 2014

the size of the reflux jet during the Valsalva maneuver. The grading is as follows:

- *Grade* 0: absence of retrograde flow.
- *Grade* 1: short reflux jet (<1 cm) with width less than 1/3 of the IJV diameter and duration inferior to 0.2 s.
- *Grade* 2: short reflux jet (<1 cm) with width less than 1/3 of the IJV diameter and duration between 0.2 and 0.4 s.
- *Grade* 3: reflux jet with width between 1/3 and 2/3 of the IJV diameter and duration greater than 0.4 s.
- *Grade* 4: reflux jet with width greater than 2/3 of the IJV diameter.

• In the majority of their studies, Chung et al. [9–12] have defined the performance modalities of the study of the jugular valve reflux as an examination that is carried out both in normal breathing conditions and during the Valsalva maneuver; the color box, in longitudinal scan, is placed with the extreme distal part located at the level of the common carotid artery flow divider. Performing the Valsalva maneuver lasts 15 s. In such a setting, the authors define as jugular reflux the presence of an inversion in the flow direction detected with color-mode and/or Doppler spectrum evaluation with a duration ≥0.5 s. However, the width of the sample volume is not specified.

• Valdueza et al. [7, 13, 14] describe a slightly different examination modality, with longitudinal scan placing the sample volume in triplex mode within the IJV at about 2 cm from the valve plane. The sample volume width is of 0.5–1 cm, and it is placed at the center of the IJV lumen. Subsequently, a Valsalva maneuver is performed with a duration greater than 5 s. In such a setting, any flow direction inversion, of whatever duration, in the Doppler spectrum during the Valsalva maneuver is considered as a reflux. The Valsalva maneuver is considered well done if the diameter of internal jugular vein increases at least 1 cm.

• Akkawi et al. [15] suggested a different evaluation modality, carried out with a 10 s Valsalva maneuver duration, before which a saline solution mixed with air (9 cc saline solution and 1 cc air) had, however, been injected intravenously. The sample volume is placed at 1.5–2 cm in a distal position with respect to the BCV. The appearance of microbubbles at the supravalvular level during the Valsalva maneuver indicates jugular valve incontinence.

• Nedelmann et al. [16, 17] standardized an evaluation methodology of the jugular valve incontinence, which also includes a time duration threshold that defines its significance. The ultrasound probe in longitudinal scan is placed on the clavicle so as to display the IJV lower bulb at the level of the confluence into the BCV. In this way, it is possible to observe the valve structures, whose closure is evaluated during a controlled Valsalva maneuver. In such a condition, the sample volume, whose dimensions are sufficient to occupy the whole width of the vessel, is placed in the IJV in close proximity to the valve apparatus (0.5 cm), and in this location, the Doppler waveform during the Valsalva maneuver is evaluated. The closure of the competent jugular valves without any sign of insufficiency is characterized by an extremely brief pre-closure venous reflux, after which the flow stops completely. When the valves are incompetent, the flow is retrograde, and clearly persistent beyond the duration of the valve closure. Valve incontinence is diagnosed on the basis of the reflux duration, >0.88 s, which signifies a value three times greater than the mean standard deviation duration of the retrograde flow of competent valves. This may help to conclusively distinguish between competent and incompetent valves, with a 100 % sensitivity and specificity.

The comparison between the method standardized by Nedelmann and colleagues, which furthermore also includes a quantitative evaluation of reflux duration, and the assessment with a shaken saline solution and gas, which also carried out by Nedelmann et al. [17], has underlined the good concordance as regards reflux identification. However, in order to avoid false negatives, it may be necessary to make the injection from the ipsilateral antecubital vein to the IJV, especially on the left, due to the length of the left BCV and of the possible phasic compressions of the sternum during the respiratory cycle. This situation may give rise to some biases.

A noteworthy element that all these evaluations have in common is the fact that all have been performed with the subject in supine position. As a result, much more information has been obtained on jugular valve incontinence in this position rather than in sitting or upright position.

The internationally accepted examination system and grading is the one standardized by Nedelmann et al. [16], and it is exemplified in the figures.

As may be well expected, the data reported in the literature vary significantly in relation to the employed methodology.

4.2 The Jugular Valve System and Valve Leaflets Malformations

In the literature, there have been only occasional reports on documented and non-controversial indications on jugular valve system alterations leading to complete anatomical stenosis or to a flow obstacle with hemodynamic consequences. In addition, such reports have been mostly carried out on patients with previous central vein catheterization or with a venous catheter inserted for a long time [18–20]. In this condition, the acquired rather than congenital nature of such a morphological trait cannot be definitely determined. Furthermore, the real hemodynamic impact is difficult to assess, due to the lack of documented normality standards to be used as comparison and to the absence of symptoms that may be correlated to such a situation.

Such findings, albeit rare, are often occasional, that is, they concern patients that have been subjected to ultrasound examinations for other reasons, such as the cases illustrated in the figures section.

4.3 The Block of Blood Flow

This finding concerns an IJV segment, inside which the blood volume is extremely small or absent, but that remains anyhow compressible. In the literature, this finding has been described in three patients affected by transient global amnesia by Chung et al. [10] in the situation of truncular reflux circuits involving the distal part of the IJV, without valves, and its branches. It was a unilateral condition of the proximal part of the IJV, temporarily regressing after a deep inspiration.

Such a finding, although being rare, has occasionally been observed in the neurosonological routine also in healthy subjects both on the right and on the left IJV. It is sometimes reversible when the head is tilted to the contra- or ipsilateral side, but at times it is non-reversible. However, this condition requires further hemodynamic elements and diagnostic tools.

4.4 Internal Jugular Vein Branches

Like the IJV, also its branches may show alterations in the expected flow direction. These flow alterations, both phasic and continuous, are related to the pressure gradient, which, however, involves J2 and J3 segments of the IJV, devoid of valves.

Incontinences of such branches may also be detected in relation to the presence of altered valve structures. Also in this case, they may be observed at rest or triggered by the Valsalva maneuver.

In the literature, some of these alterations have been documented by Chung et al. [10, 11] in a small cohort of patients with transient global amnesia as well as in healthy subjects. The evaluation was performed at rest or during deep inspiration as well as with the Valsalva maneuver; besides, the retrograde flow in the IJV branches was correlated with the presence of valve incontinence. Furthermore, in such cases, a more severe condition of venous hypertension triggered by the Valsalva maneuver was hypothesized.

4.5 Jugular Vein Thrombosis

IJV thrombosis is a rare condition but which shows a potentially severe sequel, connected both to the pulmonary embolism risk and to the intracranial propagation of the thrombus [21].

The IJV thrombosis caused by the compression of an intrathoracic goiter with an extremely slow growth is rarely described in the literature [22].

The symptoms may vary from unclear to extremely severe, including local edema of neck and face, more rarely of the superior limb. The ultrasound diagnosis is performed in a similar manner to other body locations that is by combining IJV non-compressibility in transverse scan, determined by a slight pressure of the probe, with the identification of differently echogenic material both in transverse and in longitudinal scan. The material occupies the vessel lumen and, in case of complete thrombosis, blocks the blood flow, not identifiable with Doppler mode.

There is also the possibility that the IJV ultrasound study allows to identify indirect signs of a thrombotic process localized downstream, as in the detailed example shown in the figures.

4.6 Vertebral Veins

The isolated pathology of the venous vertebral axis has not clearly been described in the literature. The ultrasound study of the cerebral venous district shows prevalently functional characteristics and must be included in a global evaluation of the cerebral and cervical venous system hemodynamics. The valve apparatus of the vertebral vein collector can be explored also morphologically with ultrasound examination [23]. Therefore, its incontinence can be identified both at rest and during the Valsalva maneuver, although neither the epidemiologic data, not its relation to pathologic conditions, are known.

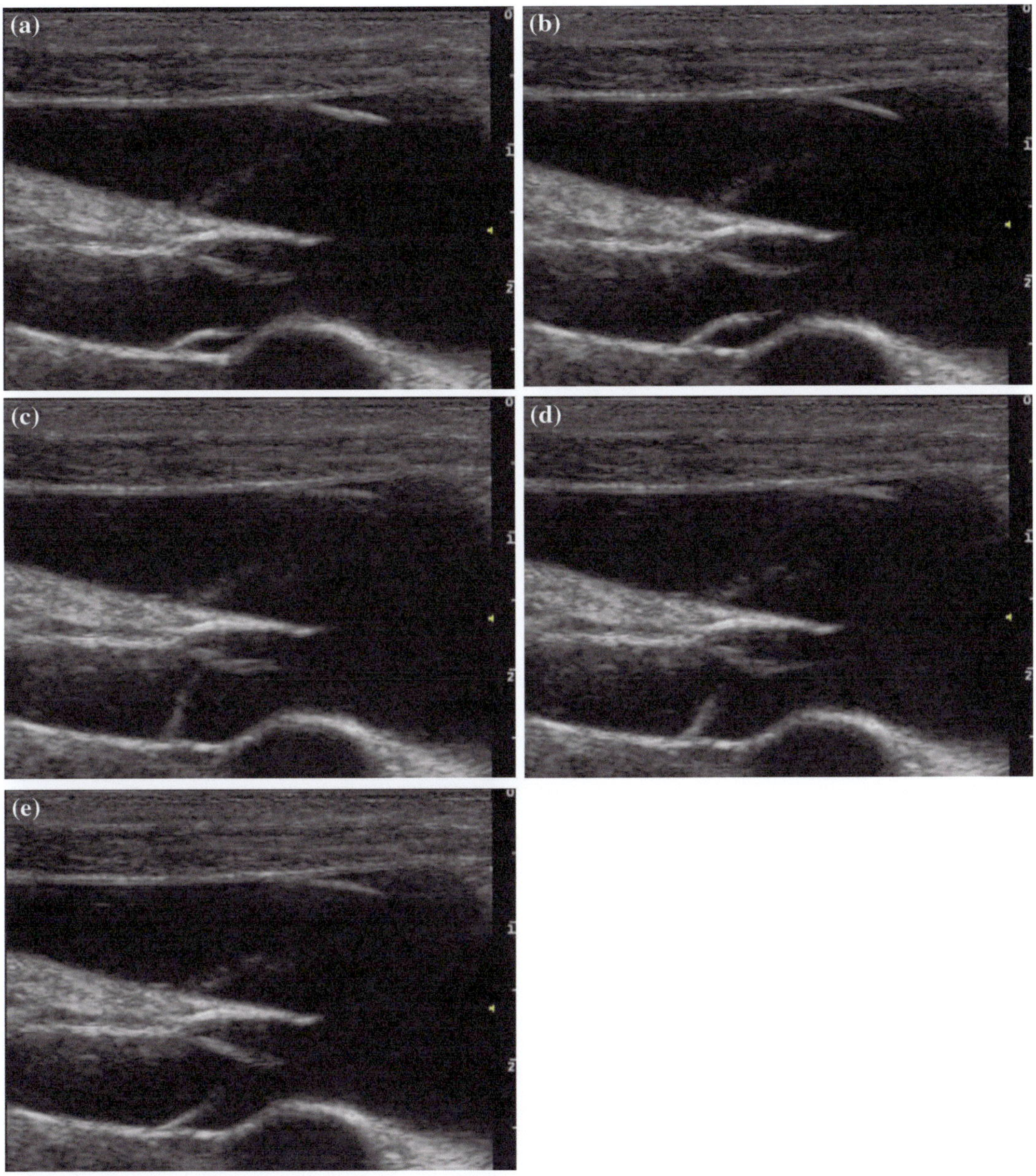

Fig. 4.1 Sequential images of the opening and closing cycle of the jugular and vertebral valve system (from **a** to **e**) as dynamically shown also in Movie 4.1. First of all, it can be noted that the IJV valve leaflets have a different length and mobility, which comes clearly across from the movie, especially regarding the upper leaflet compared to the lower one. It can also be seen that they have a dissimilar mobility as compared to the leaflets of the vertebral valve, which closes up completely by the overlapping of the leaflets (**c** and **d**), whereas the jugular valve leaflets do not seem to overlap in any phase of the cycle

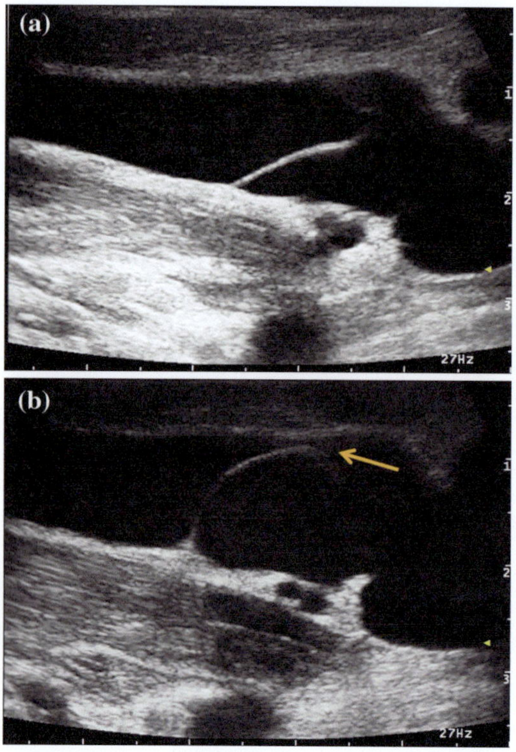

Fig. 4.2 Freeze-frame of J1 IJV during spontaneous breathing (**a**) and during Valsalva maneuver straining (**b**) in the same subject of the previous figure (see also Movie 4.2). At rest, as it clearly comes across also in the previous figure and movie, the closing of the leaflets is only occasional and not continuous with the posterior leaflet hypomobility. On the other hand, during the Valsalva maneuver, there is a perfect closure of the leaflets (*arrow*) with valve system continence. The morphological hypomobility of the lower leaflet of the IJV valve, in this case, seems to be a morphological alteration which does not seem to affect the local hemodynamics

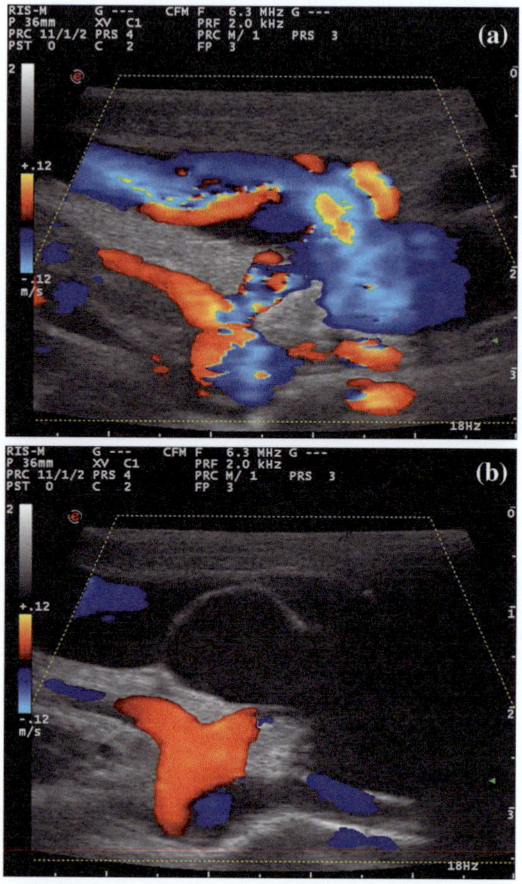

Fig. 4.3 Freeze-frame of J1 IJV during spontaneous breathing (**a**) and during Valsalva maneuver straining (**b**) in color-mode in the same subject of the previous figure (see also Movie 4.3). During spontaneous breathing, there is the confirmation of the hypomotility of the lower leaflet, which also causes a kind of preferential flow channelling along the leaflet itself, together with the laminar flow spontaneously directed toward the upper leaflet. In such a situation, the Doppler waveform will show a bidirectional flow signal, due to the mingling of two different directions of the laminar flow. However, during the Valsalva maneuver the closure of the leaflets is complete without incontinence

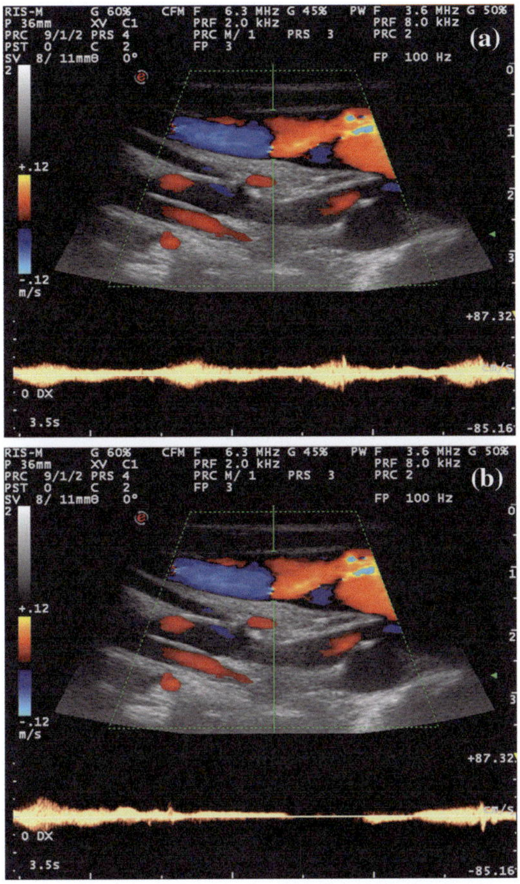

Fig. 4.4 J1 IJV in freeze-frame during spontaneous breathing (**a**) and during Valsalva maneuver straining (**b**) in the same subject of Figs. 4.1, 4.2, 4.3. At rest, note the bidirectional Doppler spectrum and the absence of incontinence during the Valsalva maneuver

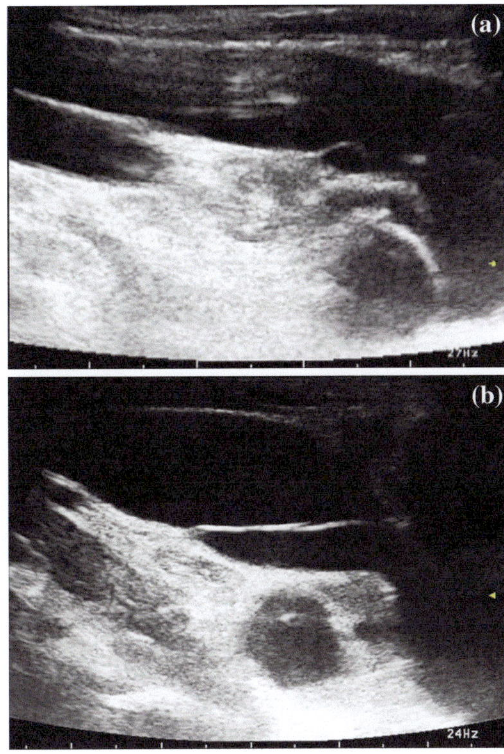

Fig. 4.5 J1 IJV longitudinal scan with two different insonation approaches: lateral (**a**), see also Movie 4.4), and anterior (**b**), see also Movie 4.5). More specifically, it is to be noted how the redundancy of the leaflets stands out in both approaches. However, if only the second approach were to be used, in this case, there would be the risk of defining the leaflets as markedly hypomobile, almost like a septum, which actually is not true

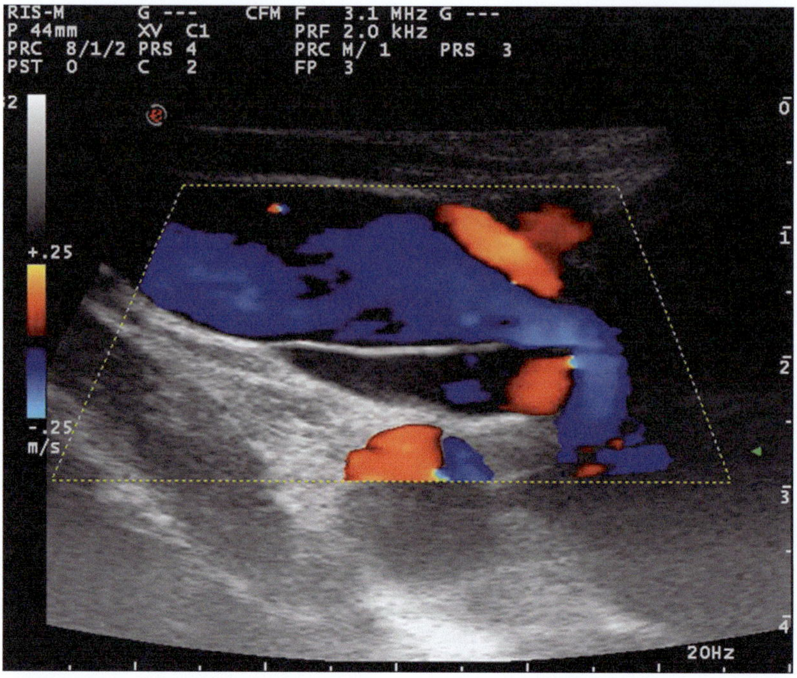

Fig. 4.6 J1 IJV color-mode longitudinal scan, with anterior approach (same subject of Fig. 4.5). As substantiation of what pointed out about the former figure, it can be noted the flow patency of the valve system (see also Movie 4.6)

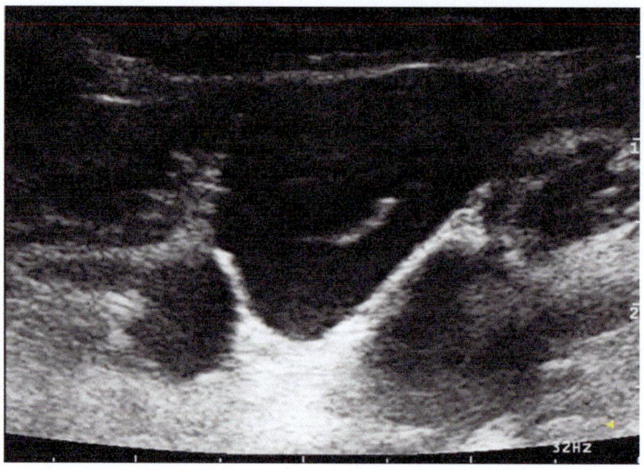

Fig. 4.7 J1 IJV transverse scan on the same subject of Figs. 4.5 and 4.6 (see also Movie 4.7). Further confirmation of the redundancy of the valve leaflets

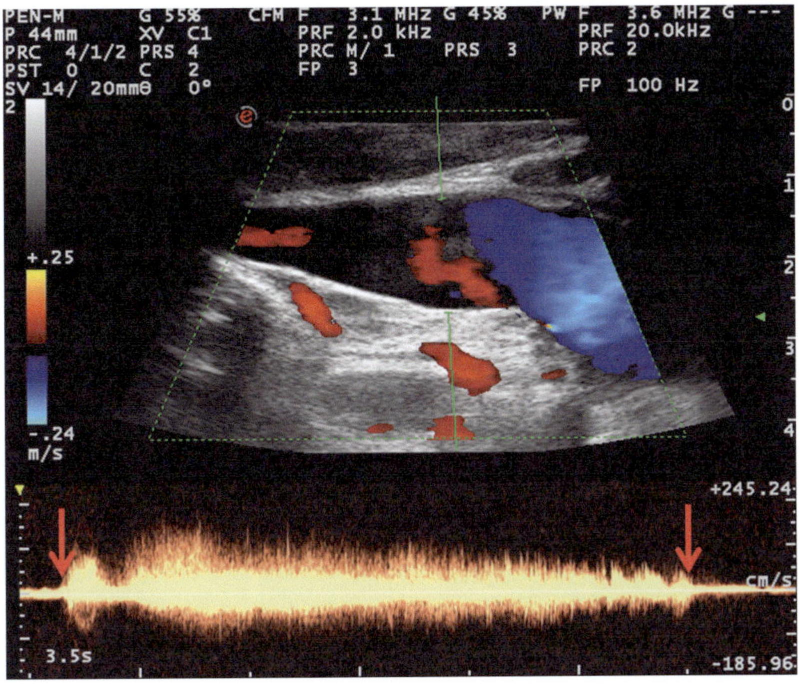

Fig. 4.8 J1 IJV color-mode longitudinal scan and corresponding Doppler waveform. Here, it is shown an example of valve incontinence caused by the Valsalva maneuver (the beginning and the end of the reflux are marked by *red arrows*) with a definitely significant duration (>2.5 s)

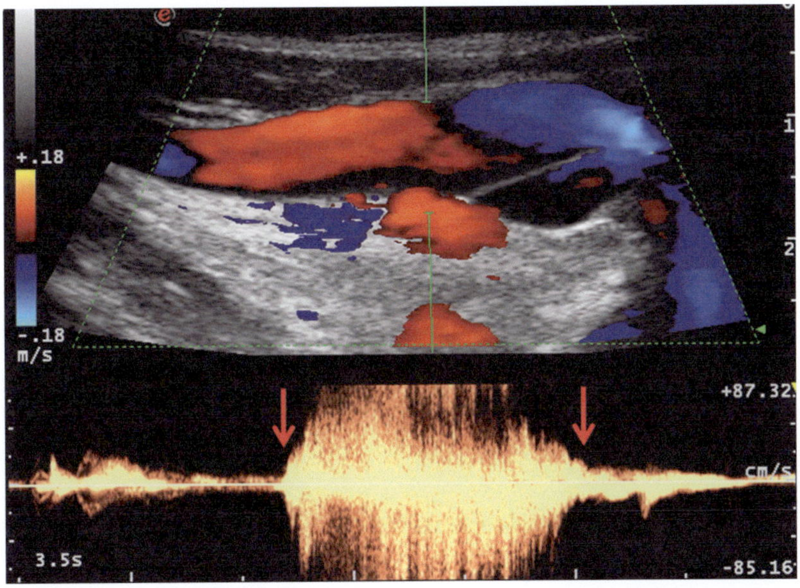

Fig. 4.9 J1 IJV color-mode longitudinal scan and corresponding Doppler waveform. Here you can see another example of valve incontinence caused by the Valsalva maneuver (the beginning and the end of the reflux are marked by *red arrows*) with a surely noteworthy duration (>1 s)

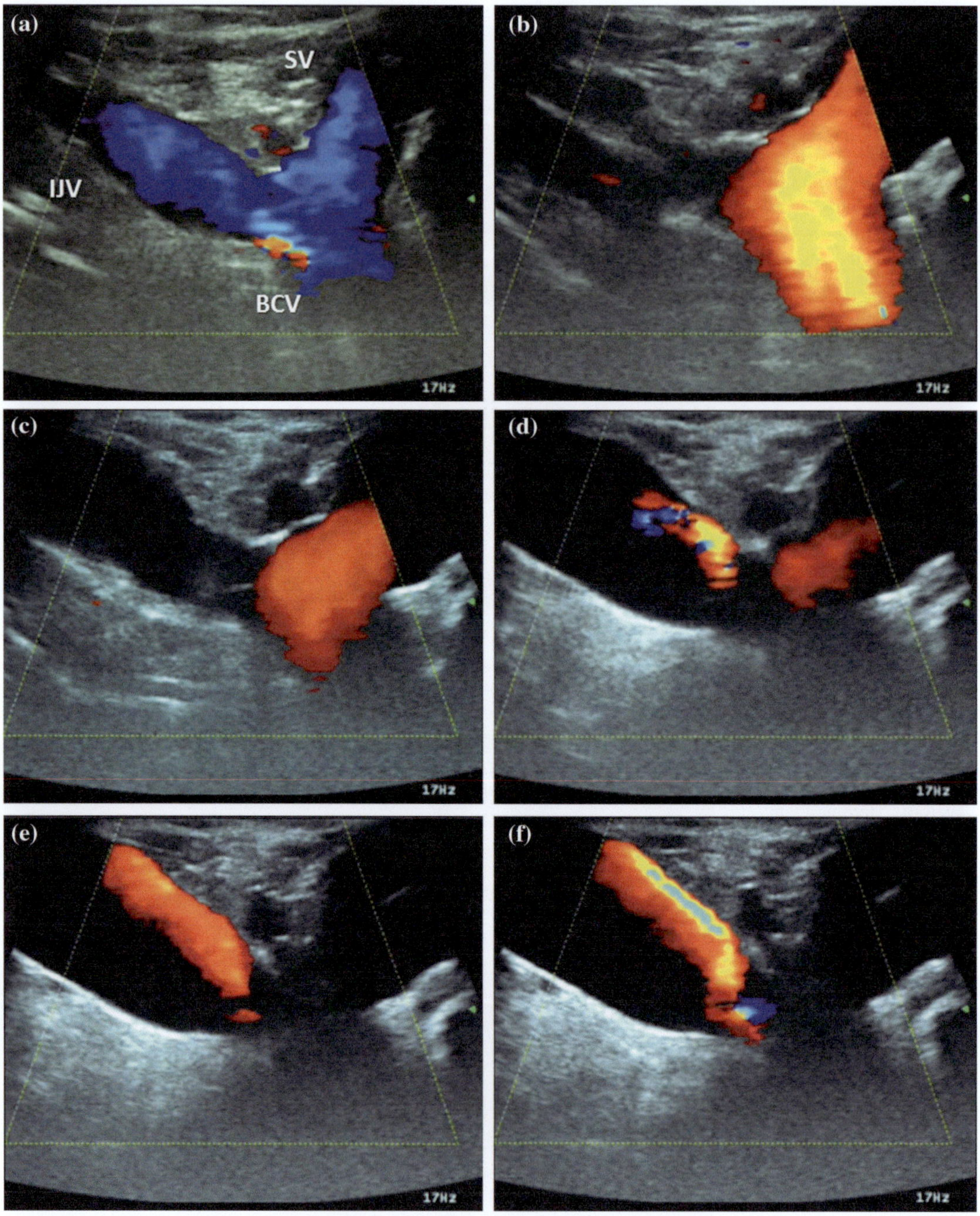

Fig. 4.10 Left IJV, subclavian access at the confluence of the SV into the BCV, color-mode. Subsequent stages during the Valsalva maneuver (Movie 4.8): **a** Pre-Valsalva inspiration, with flow in orthograde direction in IJV, SV, and BCV. **b** Initial straining phase with reflux jet on the SV and absence of flow on the IJV. **c** Intermediate straining phase, with diminishing of the reflux jet on the SV (still absence of flux in the IJV). **d** At the end of the reflux jet on the SV, initial appearance of reflux jet and aliasing on the IJV. **e** Absence of flow on SV and extension of jet on the IJV. **f** Reflux jet clearly still on IJV

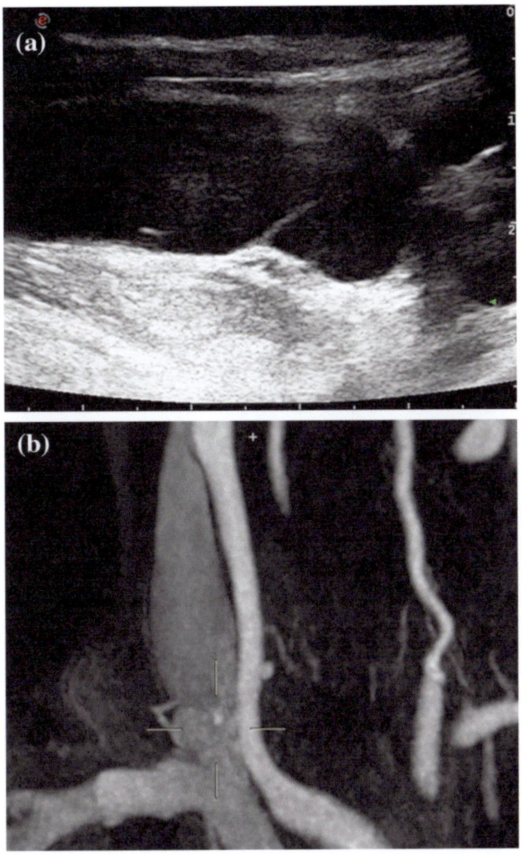

Fig. 4.11 B-mode J1 IJV longitudinal scan. IJV stenosis at the valve level. In the upper part of the picture (**a**), ultrasound image (see also Movie 4.9) that shows the fixity and distortion of the valve leaflets. In the lower part of the picture (**b**), the corresponding MR image that highlights the malformation with the stenosis at the jugular valve system level

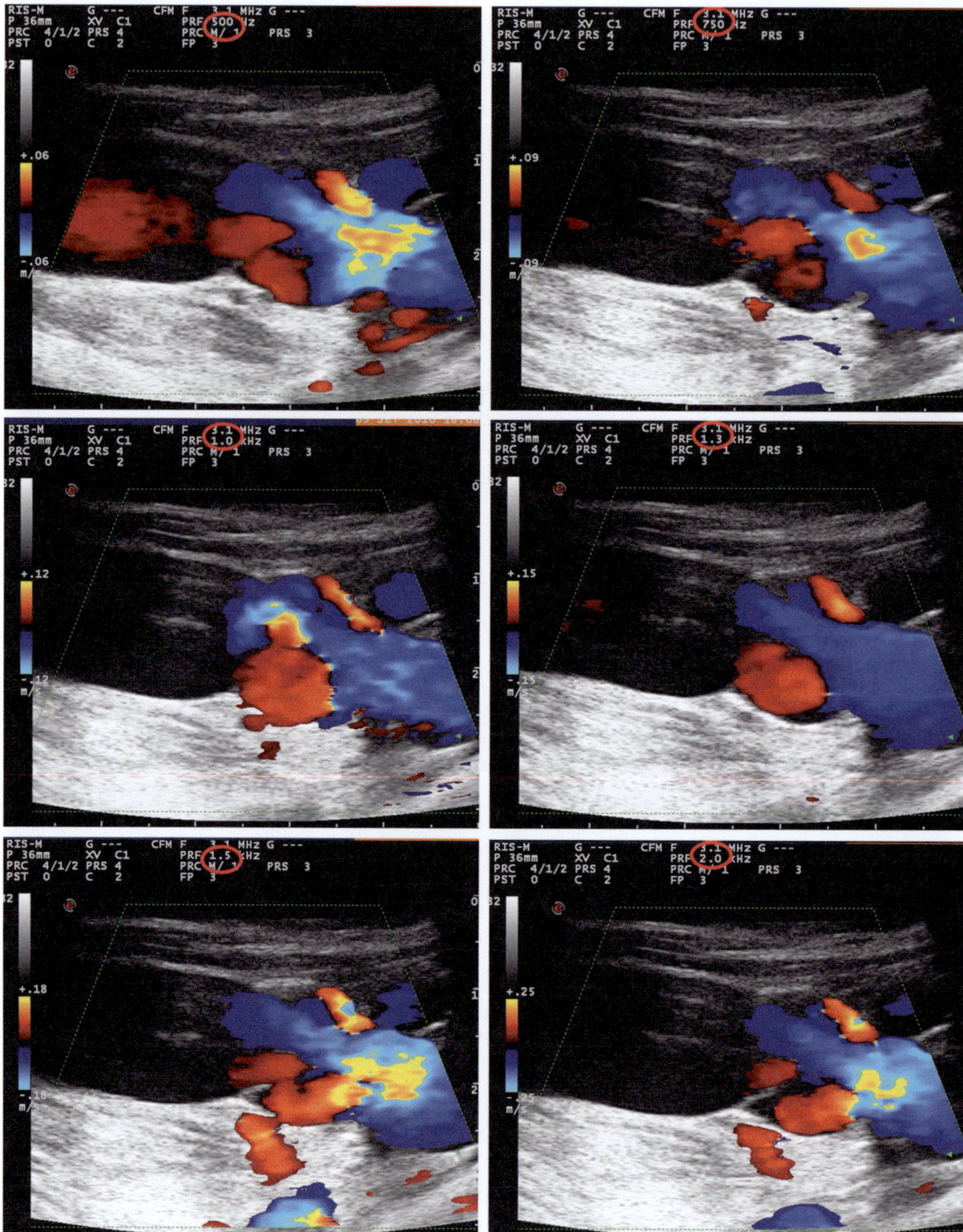

Fig. 4.12 Longitudinal scan of IJV, color mode. IJV stenosis at the valve level. In this freeze-frame image with decreasing PRF, the block of flow above the valve level is showed in color mode and the marked hypomobility of valve leaflets is well evident in the B-mode movie both at rest and with a short closure during Valsalva maneuver (see Movies 4.10, 4.11). Color-mode images and the corresponding movies: PRF decreases from 2.0 kHz to 1.5, 1.3, 1.0, 0.75, 0.5 kHz. Figure 4.12 shows the same situation illustrated in Fig. 4.11, but in color mode and zoomed on the IJV valve region. In particular, note the effect of the progressive decrease in PRF value, with equal frequency in color mode. The color signal visualization within the IJV lumen occurs only with PRF of 500 Hz, which confirms the almost complete absence of flow caused by the valve system malformation

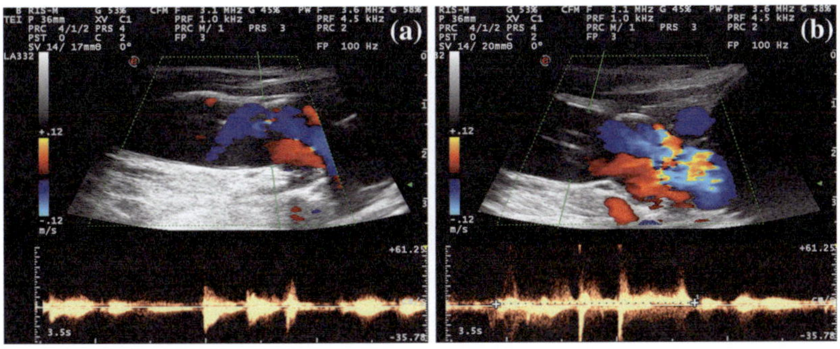

Fig. 4.13 IJV stenosis at the valve level in color mode with the Doppler waveform sampling. In figure a, the waveform in normal breathing conditions is shown; in figure b, the waveform during Valsalva maneuver marks a significant IJV valve incontinence. The valve stenosis seems a very small central hole through which the blood flow moves to and fro depending on the pressure gradient

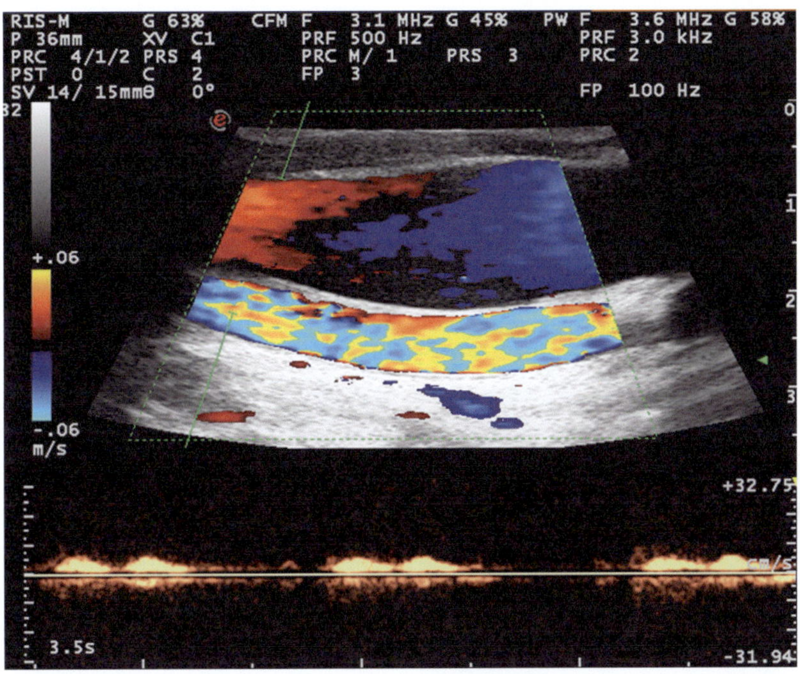

Fig. 4.14 J2 IJV segment in the same patient of the previous figures. The upstream blood flow waveform shows a phasic ≪systolic≫ flow depending on the pressure gradient, with very low velocity. The corresponding B-mode dynamic status is a spontaneous moving echo-contrast (Movie 4.12), persisting also in color mode (Movie 4.13)

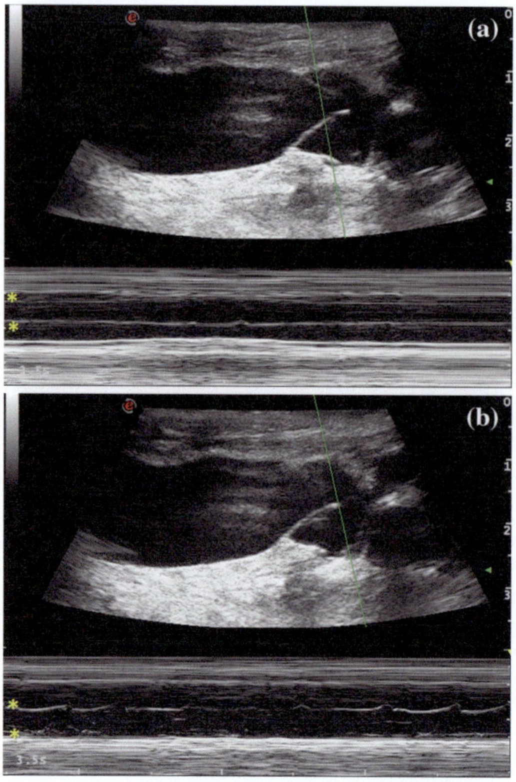

Fig. 4.15 J1 IJV of the same patient of the previous figures in M-mode (longitudinal scanning plane) at two levels of valve leaflet position. The M-line trace shows a marked hypomobility of both leaflets that remain open (*asterisk*)

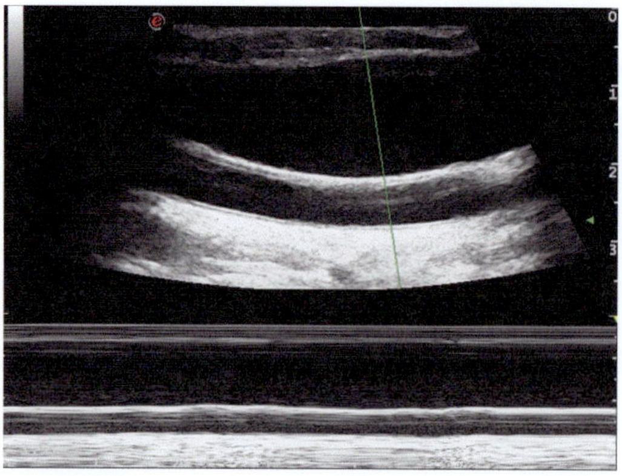

Fig. 4.16 J2 IJV segment of the same patient of the previous figures in M-mode (longitudinal scanning plane, normal breathing). A very low movement range of the wall is evident

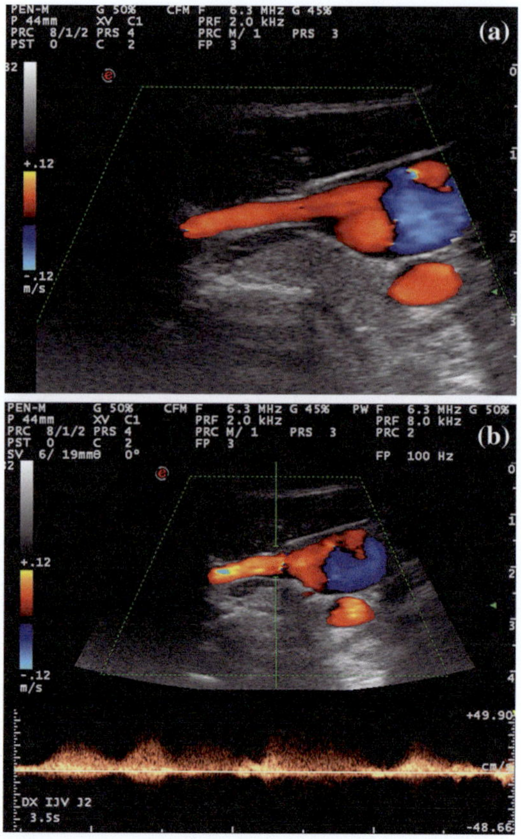

Fig. 4.17 Transverse scan of J2 IJV segment with afferent thyroid branch, during the inspiratory phase. Note how the dynamic characteristics of the afferent branch are evident and easy to study during the respiratory cycle

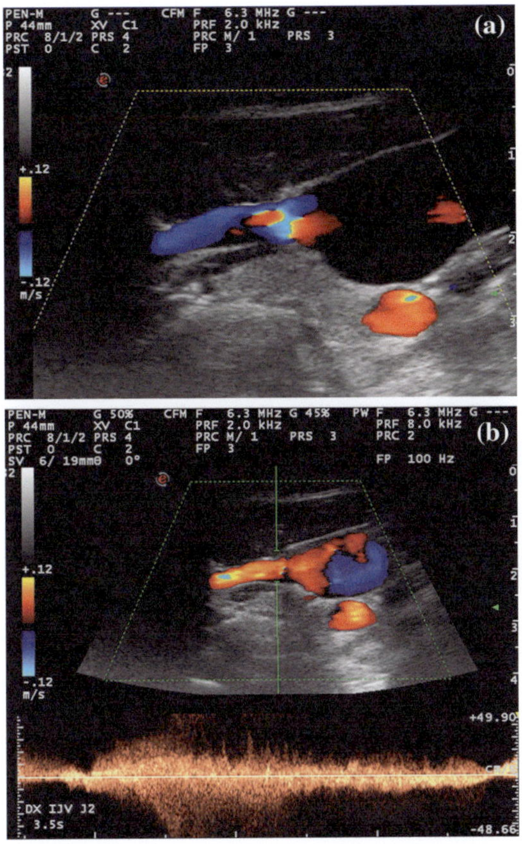

Fig. 4.18 Transverse scan of J2 IJV segment with afferent thyroid branch, during the Valsalva maneuver. Note the inversion of the flow direction in the afferent branch (**a**), whose Doppler waveform is illustrated in (**b**) (see also Movie 4.14)

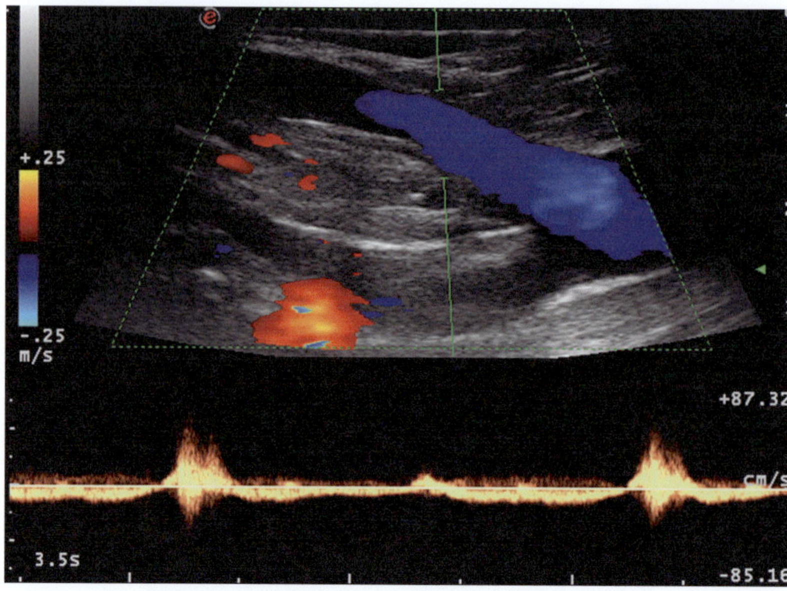

Fig. 4.19 J1 IJV longitudinal scan in a condition of venous hypoplasia. Note the Doppler waveform with the flow direction shift during normal breathing. This situation very probably indicates an incomplete valve incontinence already in basal conditions with the flow direction substantially produced by the pressure gradient without significant obstacles. As to the IJV caliber evaluation, see also Movies 4.15, 4.16

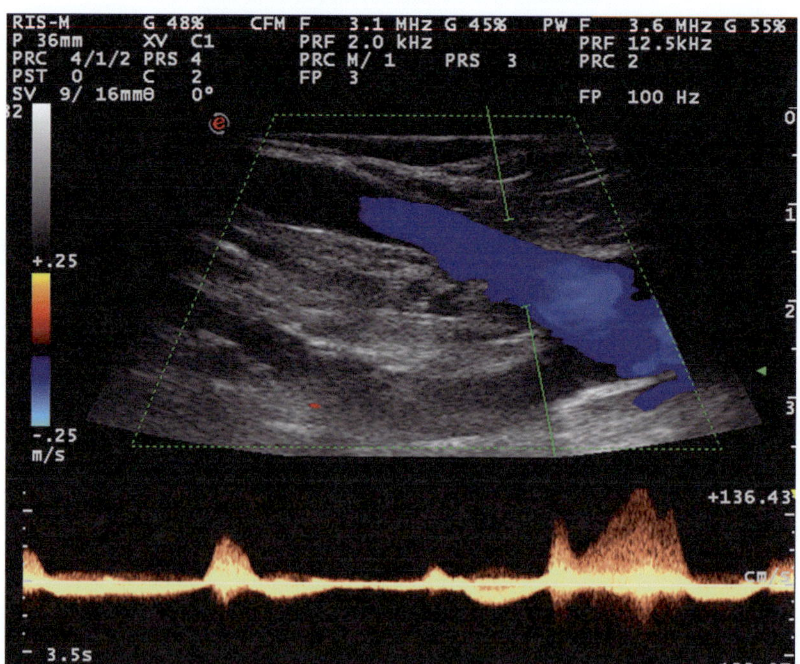

Fig. 4.20 Color-mode, J1 IJV longitudinal scan in the hypoplastic vein. In this situation, the performing of the Valsalva maneuver causes a temporary, although not significant, increase in the duration of the jet reflux

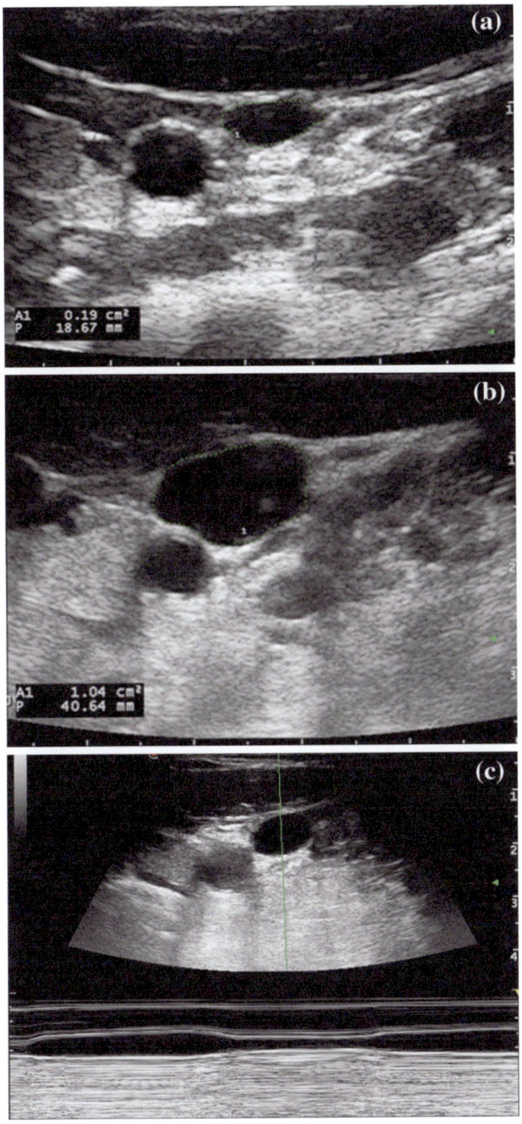

Fig. 4.21 J2 IJV, hypoplastic vein, the same subject of the former figure. In picture a, the J2 IJV CSA can be evaluated. It is decidedly reduced as expected, but it is consistent with what is described in the literature, regarding the IJV size asymmetry between one side and the other. As a comparison, in picture b, the contralateral J2 IJV area has been marked. Picture c, in M-mode, transverse access, as in Movie 4.17, a wide range of the vein caliber, connected with the respiratory cycle, is highlighted

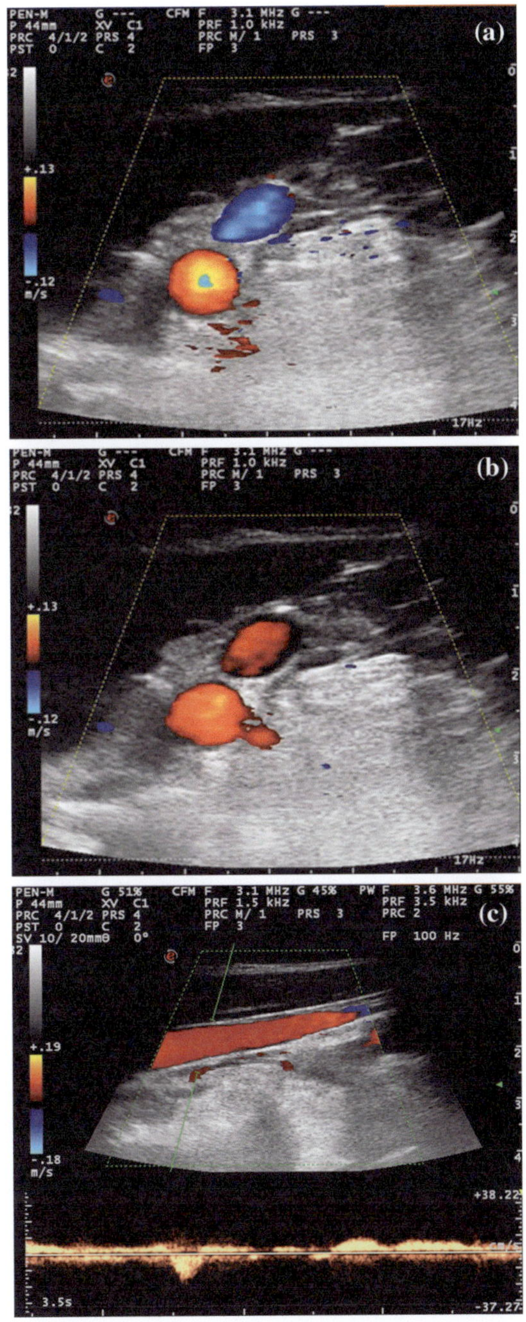

Fig. 4.22 J2 IJV, hypoplastic vein. Same subject of the previous figure. In the upper row, J2 IJV can be seen in color-mode transverse scan, **a** during the inspiratory phase and **b** in the expiratory phase. It can be noted how the flow direction is opposite in the two respiratory phases, since it is retrograde during the expiratory phase (see also Movie 4.18). The picture **c** also illustrates the corresponding Doppler waveform, in longitudinal scan, which shows a similar shift in the flow direction

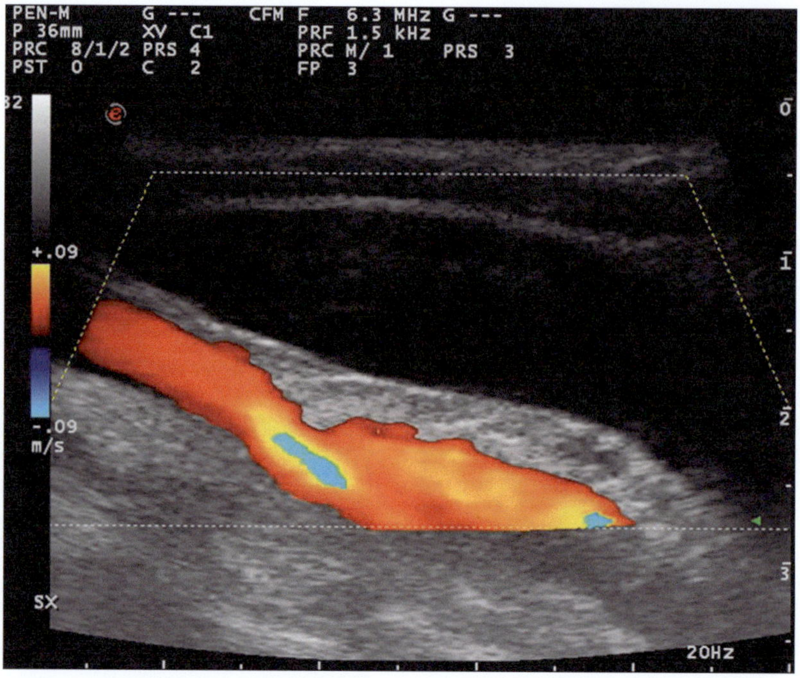

Fig. 4.23 Color-mode, longitudinal scan of J1-2 IJV. The outstanding element is the absence of the color-coded filling of the IJV lumen, as if the flow was absent or the lumen empty. See also corresponding Movie 4.19

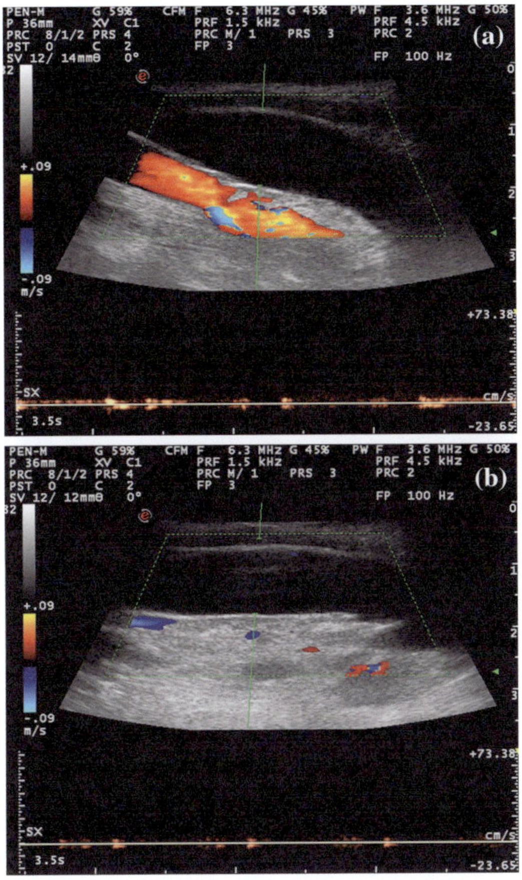

Fig. 4.24 J1-2 IJV in color mode with Doppler waveform in two different positions (**a** in neutral position of the neck and **b** with contralateral tilting of about 30°). The most evident feature is the absence of colorimetric filling of the IJV lumen with associated Doppler waveform characterized by the absence of flow, with patent and well-compressible lumen of the vessel (see Movie 4.20)

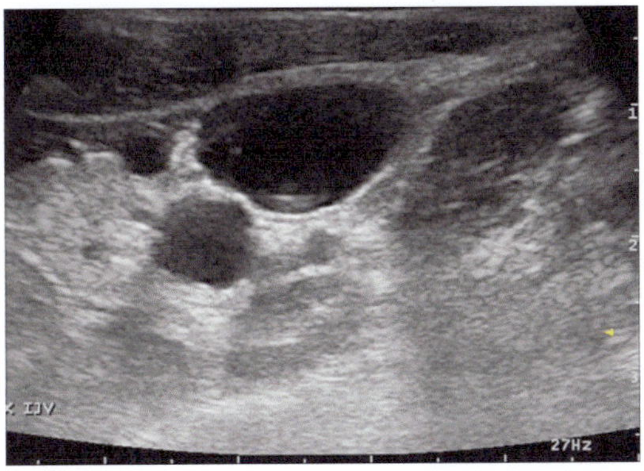

Fig. 4.25 J2 IJV, B-mode, transverse scan. The most evident element is the particulate content, finely hyperechoic, of the IJV lumen, which, however, is patent and well compressible, and corresponds to the spontaneous echo-contrast associated with the flow stasis

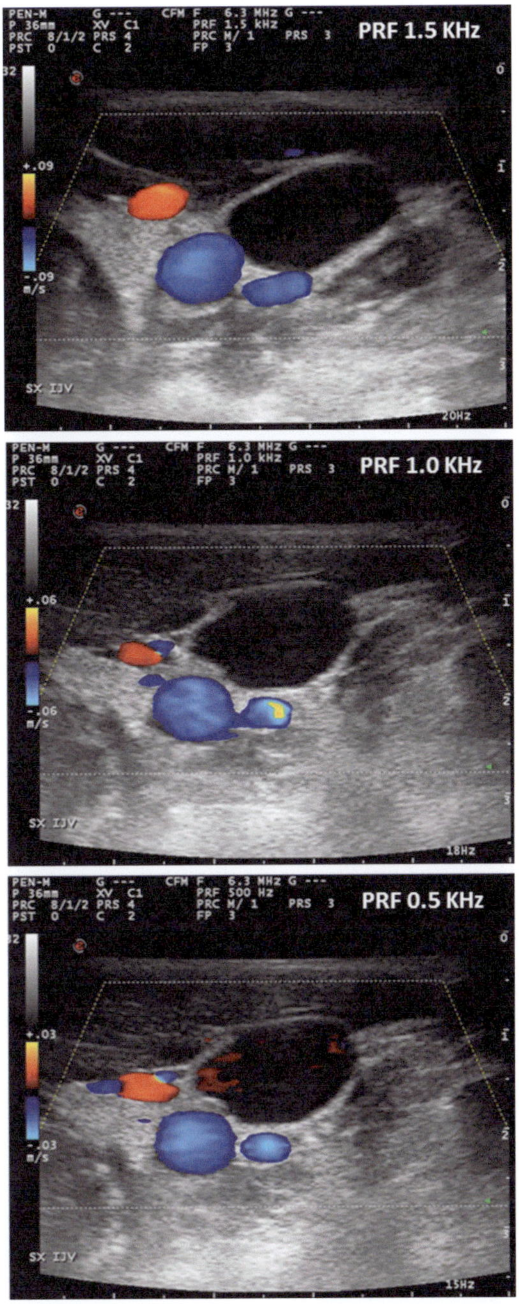

Fig. 4.26 B-mode, J2 IJV in color-mode transverse scan. The most significant feature is the fact that, despite the progressive decrease of PRF (*top* to *bottom* in the pictures, with the indication of the single value in *top-right corner*), not even a minimal colorimetric spot within the lumen can be detected, unless with PRF 0.5 kHz. See also the corresponding Movies 4.22, 4.23, 4.24

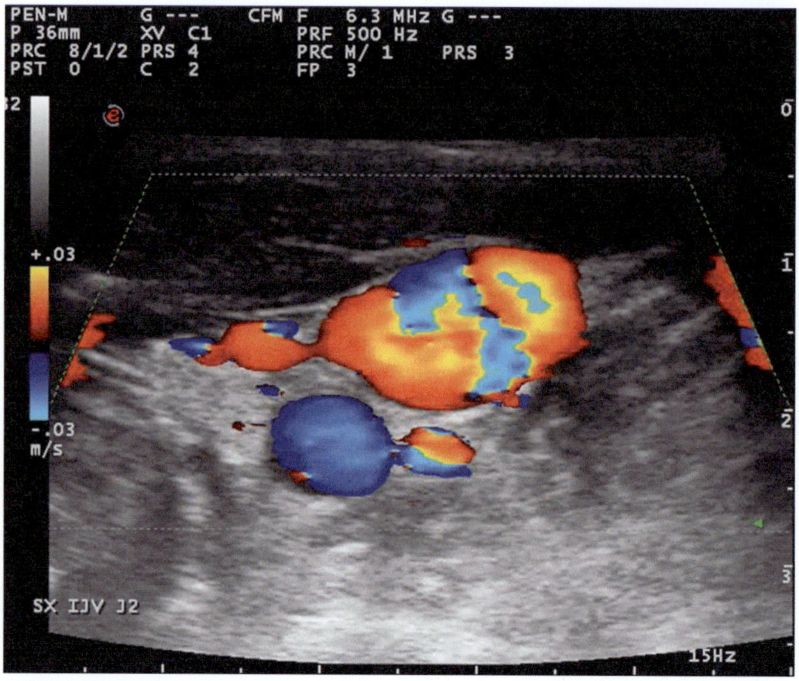

Fig. 4.27 B-mode, J2 IJV transverse scan in color mode during Valsalva maneuver. Only during the straining phase of the Valsalva maneuver, although in a transient way, it is possible to mark the presence of a flow inside the lumen vessel. This is a further confirmation of its patency. See also the corresponding Movie 4.25

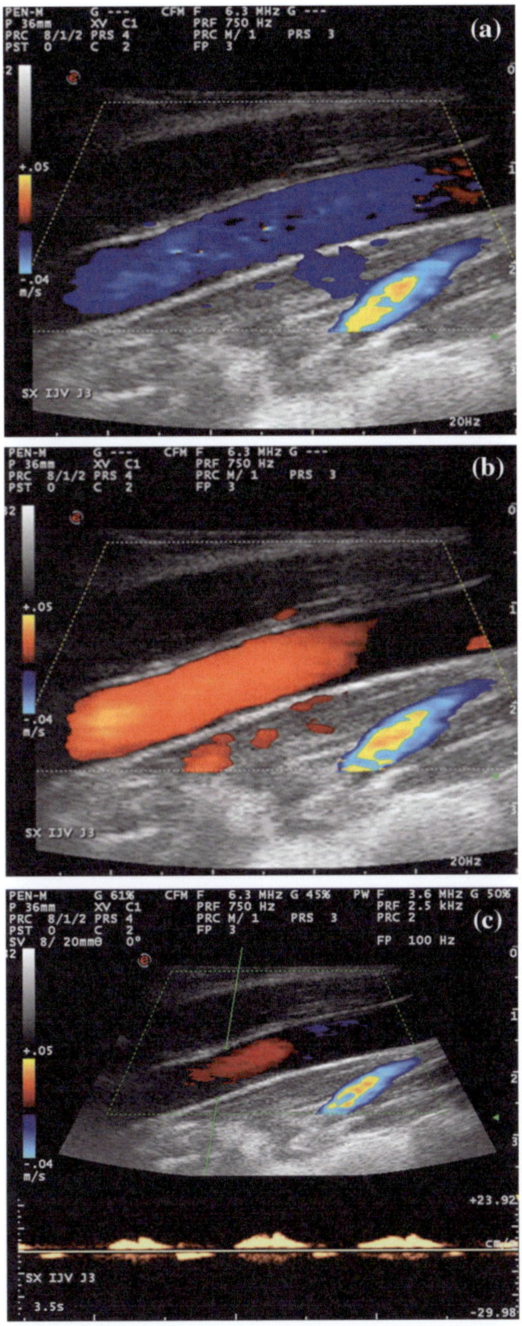

Fig. 4.28 B-mode and color-mode J3 IJV longitudinal scan (same subject of Figs. 4.22, 4.23, 4.24, 4.25, 4.26, 4.27). On the *top-left* (a), the inversion of flow direction during the expiratory phase is shown, whereas the direction is orthograde in the inspiratory phase (**b**) (see also Movies 4.26, 4.27). In the *bottom* picture (**c**), there is a Doppler waveform evaluation, which corroborates what was highlighted in color mode, with the alternating flow direction in the respiratory cycle phases

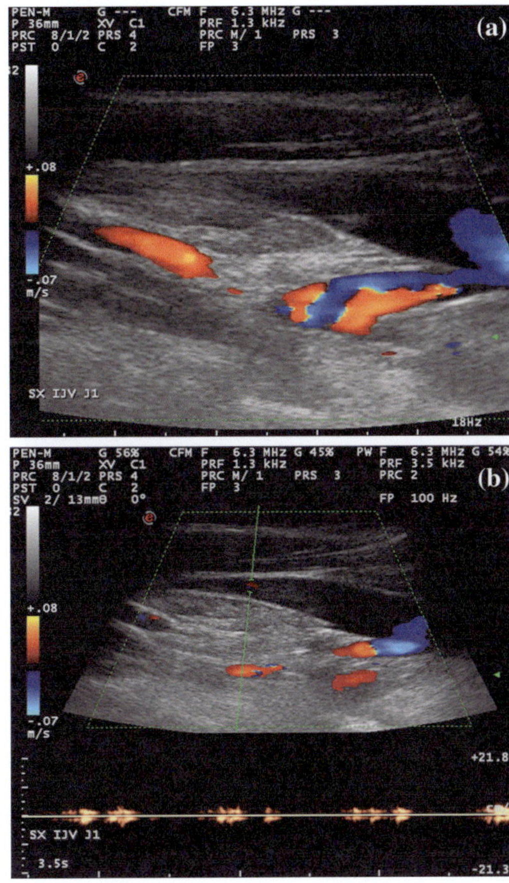

Fig. 4.29 Color-mode, J1 IJV longitudinal scan in upright position. The top picture (**a**) shows color-mode image, with a manifest absence of colorimetric filling of IJV (on the contrary, VV filling is present) (see also Movie 4.28). In the bottom picture (**b**), there is a Doppler waveform evaluation, which confirms the data highlighted in color mode, with flow signal absence

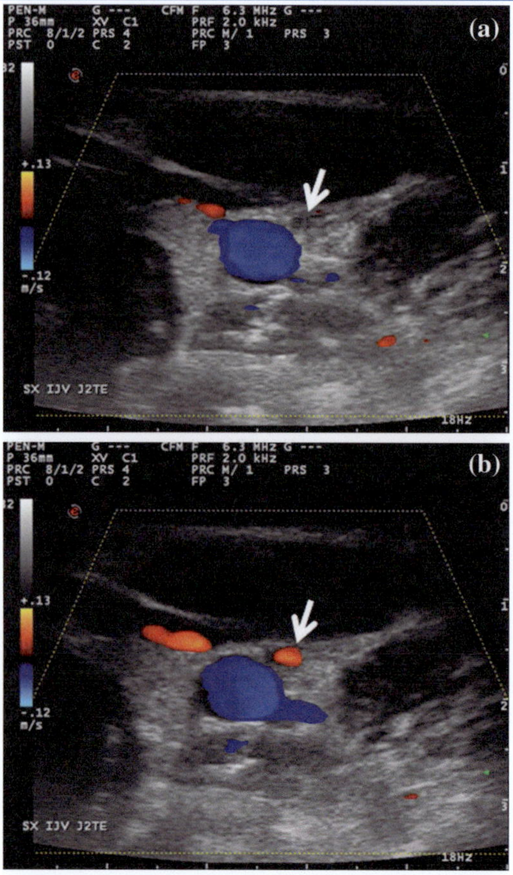

Fig. 4.30 Color-mode, J2 IJV transverse scan in orthostatic position. Picture (**a**) shows normal breathing conditions with a difficult identification of the IJV empty lumen. Picture (**b**) shows deep inspiration, with orthograde flow on JIV (see also Movie 4.29). J2 IJV is indicated with a *white arrow*

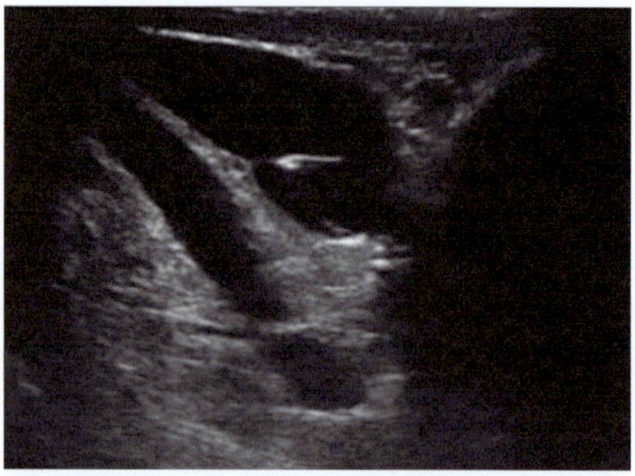

Fig. 4.31 B-mode, J1 IJV longitudinal scan. Both in the still image and in the movies (Movies 4.30, 4.31), at the level of the valve sinuses, a series of hyperechoic dot-like signals can be detected. They correspond to a hypomobile leaflet. In the movie, they are whirling and they can no longer be seen during the Valsalva maneuver. This pattern refers to stasis, slowing down and local whirling movement of the blood flow

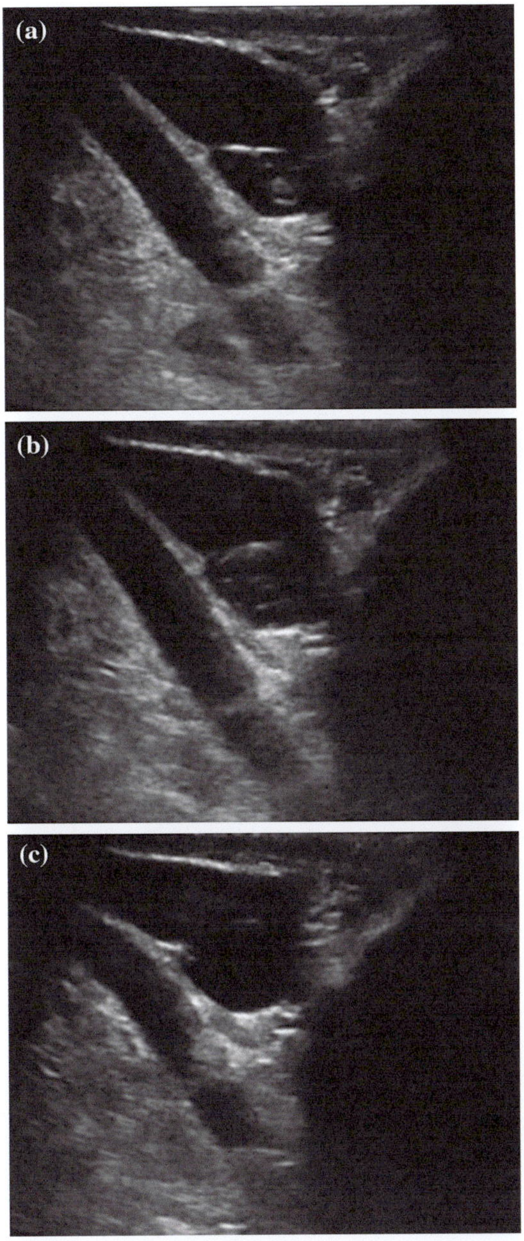

Fig. 4.32 B-mode, J1 IJV longitudinal scan. Three subsequent freeze-frames concerning the end of the inspiratory pre-Valsalva phase (pictures **a** and **b**) and at the beginning of the Valsalva maneuver (picture **c**). By stopping the flow produced by the Valsalva maneuver, the disappearance of the spontaneous echo-contrast at the level of the valve sinus can be observed (see Movie 4.31)

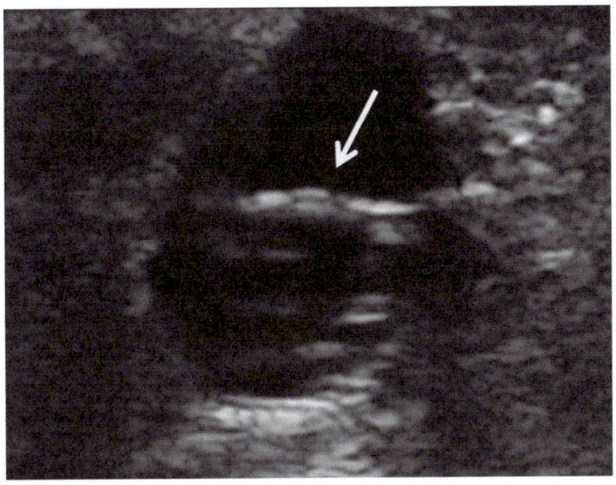

Fig. 4.33 B-mode, J1 IJV in axial scan (*magnified image*). The middle of the picture shows the valve leaflets in the closure phase (*white arrow*). At the level of the lower valve sinus, there is a marked spontaneous echo-contrast (see Movie 4.32)

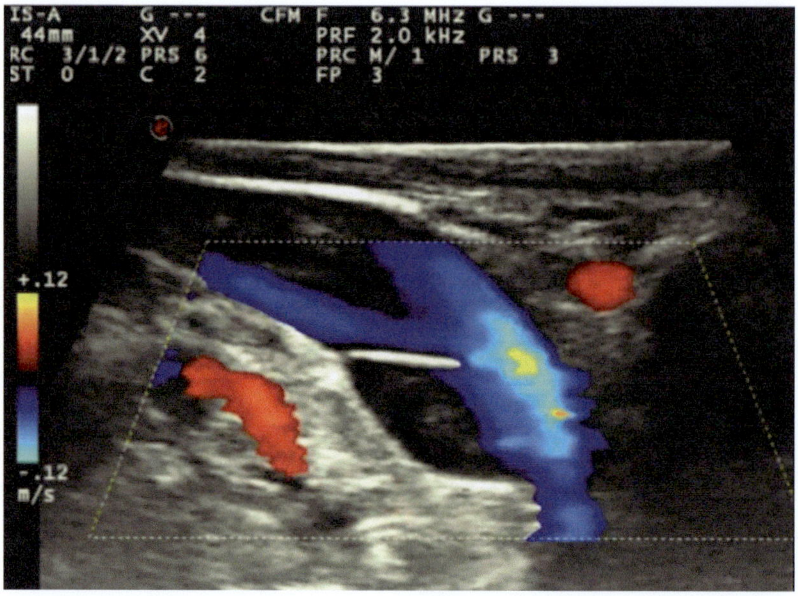

Fig. 4.34 Color-mode, J1 IJV longitudinal scan. Both the still image and the movie (Movie 4.33) highlight a clear spontaneous echo-contrast at the level of the valve sinus corresponding to the posterior hypomobile leaflet. This region is rarely covered by the colorimetric filling, and this indicates a lower velocity in that position that can be attributed to local stasis of the blood flow

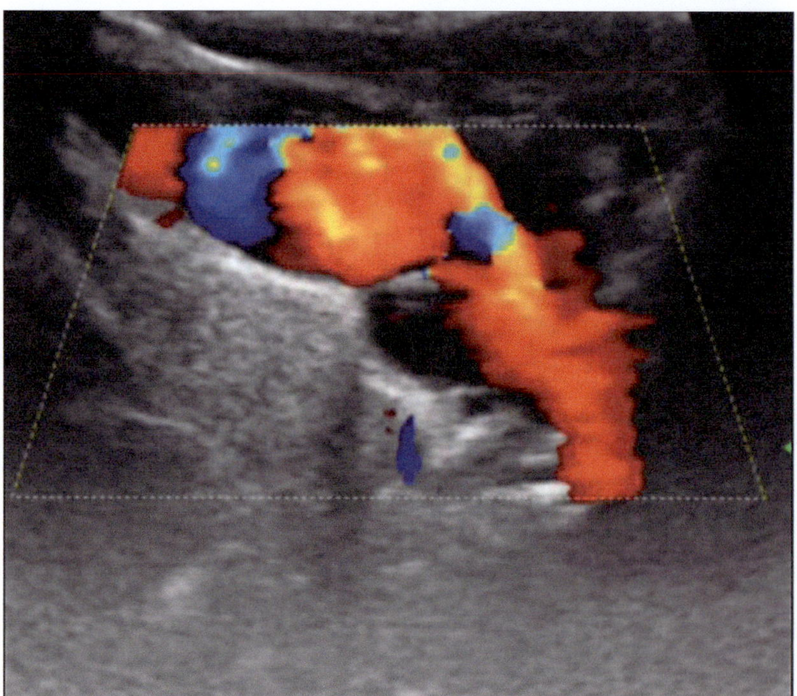

Fig. 4.35 Color-mode, J1 IJV longitudinal scan. The Valsalva maneuver produces an eccentric valve incontinence with simultaneous hypomobility of the posterior valve leaflet. This incontinence is caused by the failed closure of the anterior leaflet (Movie 4.34)

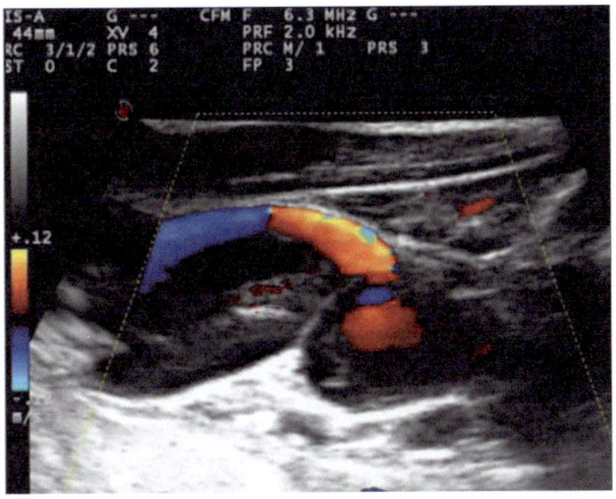

Fig. 4.36 Color-mode, J1 IJV in longitudinal scan, with anterior access. With an anterior access, during Valsalva maneuver straining, the eccentric position of the reflux jet stands out even more clearly. However, it is also present in normal breathing conditions, but it is phasic and has shorter duration (see the next figure and Movie 4.35)

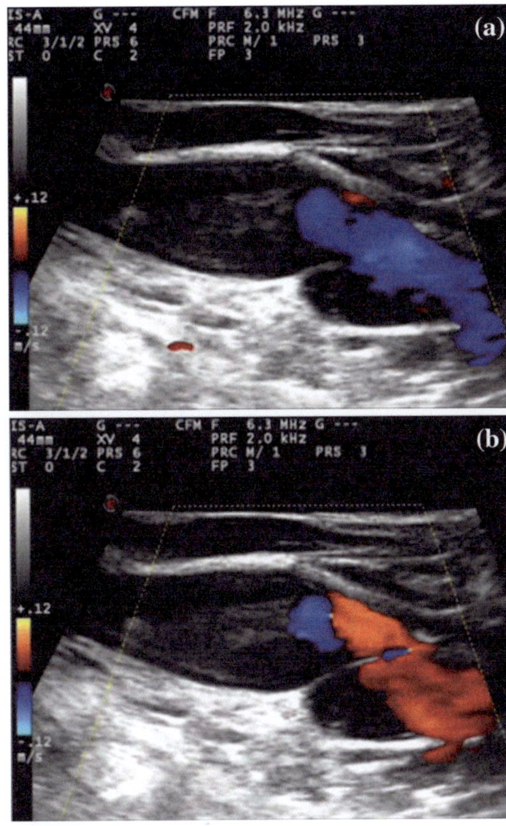

Fig. 4.37 Color-mode, J1 IJV longitudinal scan, with anterior access, in normal breathing conditions. The picture on the *left* illustrates a normal flow direction in the IJV during the inspiratory phase, while the picture on the *right* shows the expiratory phase, with phasic inversion of the flow direction (see Movie 4.35)

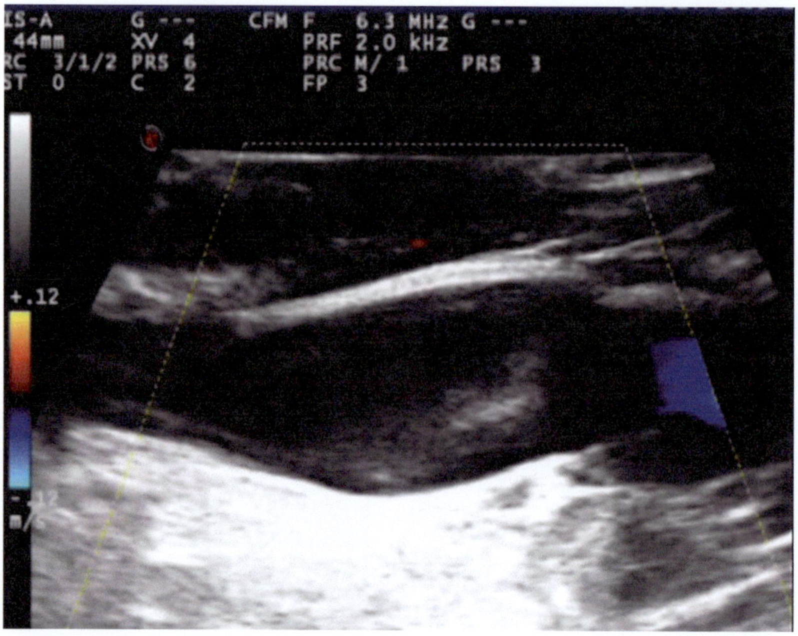

Fig. 4.38 Color-mode, J1 IJV longitudinal scan, anterior access, during spontaneous breathing. At the level of the jugular bulb, the marked spontaneous echo-contrast can be noticed, with little colorimetric filling (see Movie 4.36)

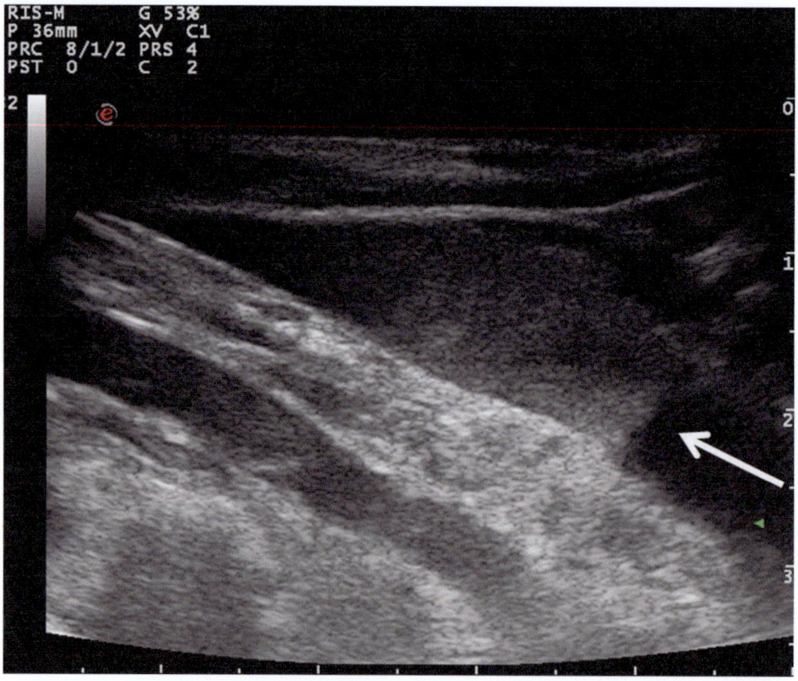

Fig. 4.39 B-mode, J1 IJV longitudinal scan. It clearly comes across that the IJV lumen is quite entirely filled with finely hyperechoic material, which ends at the level of the valve plane with a sort of "meniscus" (*white arrow*) (see Movie 4.37). The patient under examination suffered from venous thrombosis of the SV-BCV junction, which very probably was the cause of an extremely marked stasis at the level of the IJV J1, with an endoluminal spontaneous echo-contrast. This situation must be distinguished from a local thrombotic process, which in the acute phase may be dislocated by the probe pressure, thus producing a CUS with a false negative result

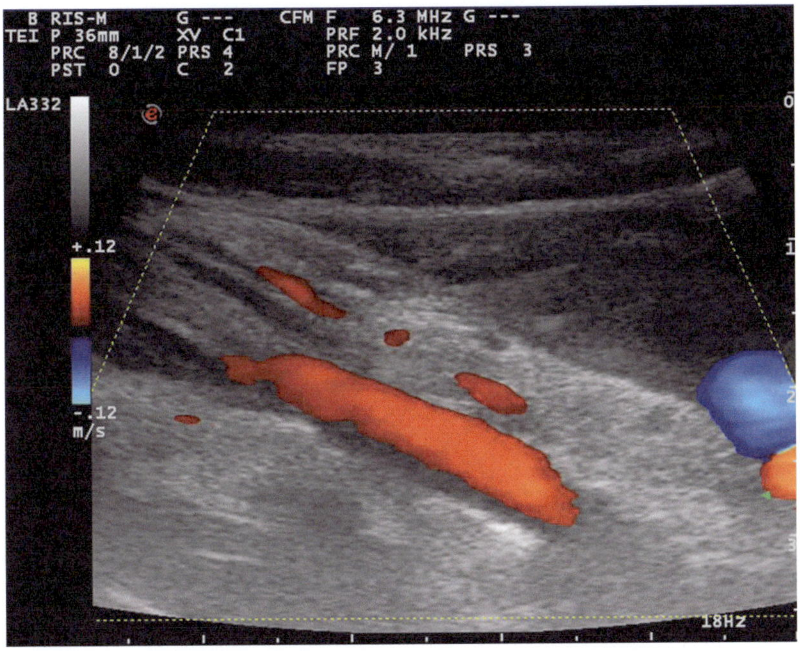

Fig. 4.40 Color-mode, J1 IJV longitudinal scan. The subject is the same of the previous picture, and it clearly shows how the IJV lumen, almost entirely filled with finely echogenic material, which is, however, mobile (see Movie 4.38), corresponds to a segment not filled by moving blood. Transverse scan in caudo-cranial direction (Movie 4.39): the supravalvular segment is fully compressible. This feature is less easy to evaluate at the valve level on account of the position of the junction

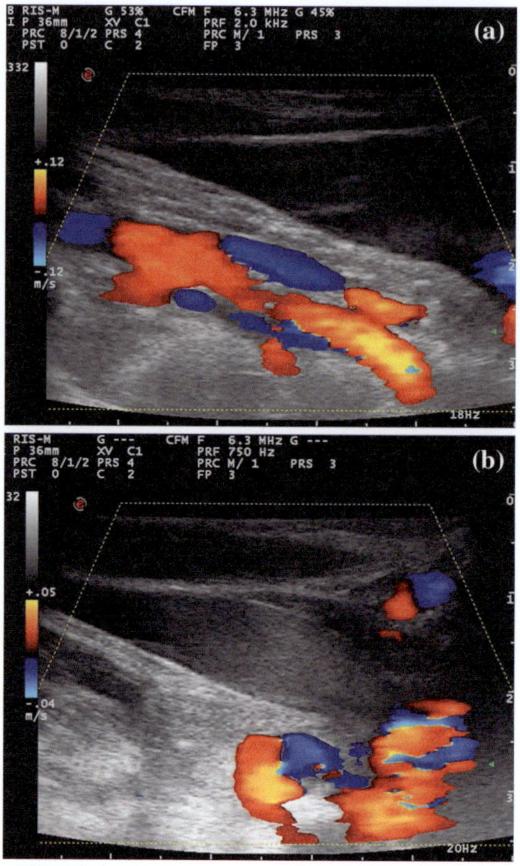

Fig. 4.41 Color-mode, J1 IJV in longitudinal scan. The lack of lumen filling can clearly be observed with different settings, especially in figure **a** with PRF 2 kHz (see Movie 4.40) and in figure **b** with PRF 0.75 kHz (see Movie 4.41)

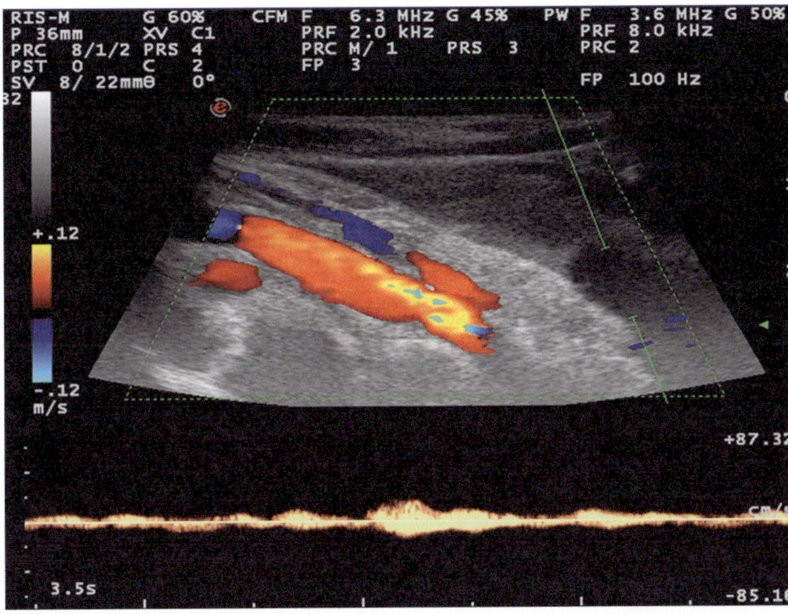

Fig. 4.42 Color-mode, J1 IJV in longitudinal scan with Doppler spectrum. It clearly comes across how the Doppler waveform, sampled in the most proximal point where it is possible to find the flow, i.e., at the level of the directly subvalvular plane of the IJV, shows a bidirectional flow waveform of extremely low velocity

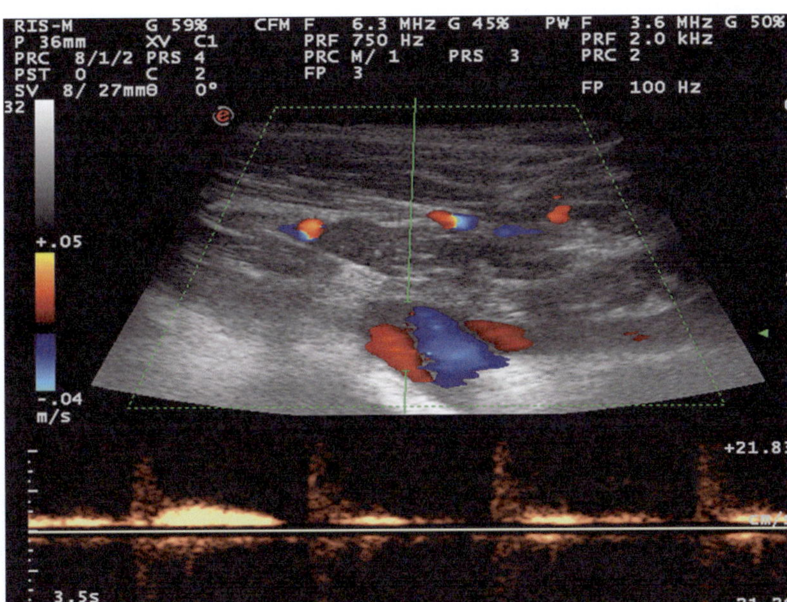

Fig. 4.43 Color-mode, SV in supraclavear access with Doppler waveform. The proximal SV, involved in the thrombotic process, shows a similar Doppler waveform

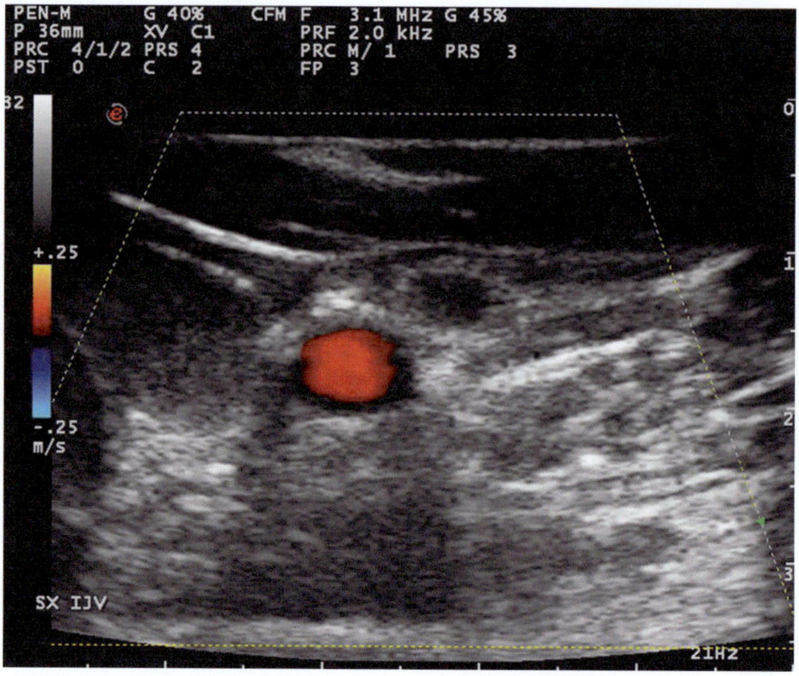

Fig. 4.44 Color-mode, IJV J2 in transverse access. In this situation, the absence of flow inside the lumen, occupied by hyperechoic material, stands out as direct evidence of the jugular vein thrombosis. On the contrary, the flow signal at the level of the common carotid artery is well evident. In Movie 4.42, the lack of IJV compressibility at CUS can be observed

References

1. Dresser LP, McKinney WM (1987) Anatomic and pathophysiologic studies of the human internal jugular valve. Am J Surg 154:220–224
2. Paradis NA, Martin GB, Goetting MG, Rosenberg JM, Rivers EP, Appleton TJ, Nowak RM (1989) Simultaneous aortic, jugular bulb, and right atrial pressures during cardiopulmonary resuscitation in humans: Insights into mechanisms. Circulation 80:361–368
3. Chung C-P, Hsu H-Y, Chao A-C, Chang F-C, Sheng W-Y, Hu H-H (2006) Detection of intracranial venous reflux in patients of transient global amnesia. Neurology 66:1873–1877
4. Akkawi NM, Agosti C, Anzola GP, Borroni B, Magoni M, Pezzini A, Rozzini L, Vignolo LA, Padovani A (2003) Transient global amnesia: a clinical and sonographic study. Eur Neurol 49:67–71
5. Nedelmann M, Eicke BM, Dieterich M (2005) Increased incidence of jugular valve insufficiency in patients with transient global amnesia. J Neurol 252:1482–1486
6. Sander D, Winbeck K, Etgen T, Knapp R, Klingelhofer J, Conrad B (2000) Disturbance of venous flow patterns in patients with transient global amnesia. Lancet 356:1982–1984
7. Schreiber SJ, Doepp F, Klingebiel R, Valdueza JM (2005) Internal jugular vein valve incompetence and intracranial venous anatomy in transient global amnesia. J Neurol Neurosurg Psychiatry 76:509–513
8. Wu X, Studer W, Erb T, Skarvan K, Seeberger MD (2000) Competence of the internal jugular vein valve is damaged by cannulation and catheterization of the internal jugular vein. Anesthesiology 93(2):319–324
9. Wu IH, Sheng WY, Hu HH, Chung CP (2011) Jugular venous reflux could influence cerebral blood flow: a transcranial Doppler study. Acta Neurol Taiwan 20:15–21
10. Chung CP, Hsu HY, Chao AC, Sheng WY, Soong BW, Hu HH (2007) Transient global amnesia: cerebral venous outflow impairment-insight from the abnormal flow patterns of the internal jugular vein. Ultrasound Med Biol 33(11):1727–1735
11. Chung CP, Hsu HY, Chao AC, Wong WJ, Sheng WY, Hu HH (2007) Flow volume in the jugular vein and related hemodynamics in the branches of the jugular vein. Ultrasound Med Biol 33(4):500–505
12. Chung CP, Lin YJ, Chao AC, Lin SJ, Chen YH, Wang YJ, Hu HH (2010) Jugular venous hemodynamic changes with aging. Ultrasound Med Biol 36(11):1776–1782

13. Doepp F, Valdueza JM, Schreiber SJ (2007) Incompetence of internal jugular valve in patients with primary. Cephalalgia 28:182–185
14. Doepp F, Valdueza JM, Schreiber SJ (2008) Incompetence of internal jugular valve in patients with primary exertional headache: a risk factor?, Cephalalgia 28(2):182–185. Epub 2007 Nov 16
15. Akkawi NM, Agosti C, Borroni B, Rozzini L, Magoni M, Vignolo LA, Padovani A (2002) Jugular valve incompetence. A study using air contrast ultrasonography on a general population. J Ultrasound Med 21:747–751
16. Nedelmann M, Eicke BM, Dieterich M (2005) Functional and morphological criteria of internal jugular valve insufficiency as assessed by ultrasound. J Neuroimaging 15:70–75
17. Nedelmann M, Teschner D, Dieterich M (2007) Analysis of internal jugular vein insufficiency—a comparison of two ultrasound methods. Ultrasound Med Biol 33(6):857–862
18. Oguzkurt L, Tercan F, Yildirim S, Torun D (2005) Central venous stenosis in haemodialysis patients without a previous history of catheter placement. Eur J Radiol 55:237–242
19. Taal MW, Chesterton LJ, McIntyre CW (2004) Venography at insertion of tunnelled internal jugular vein dialysis catheters reveals significant occult stenosis. Nephrol Dial Transplant 19:1542–1545
20. MacRae JM, Ahmed A, Johnson N, Levin A, Kiaii M (2005) Central vein stenosis: a common problem in patients on hemodialysis. ASAIO J 51:77–81
21. Sheikh MA, Topoulos AP, Deitcher SR (2002) Isolated internal jugular vein thrombosis: risk factors and natural history. Vasc Med 7(3):177–179
22. Marcelino M, Nobre E, Conceição J, Lopes L, Vilar H, De Castro JJ (2010) Superior vena cava syndrome and substernal goiter. Thyroid 20(2):235–236
23. Chou CH, Chao AC, Hu HH (2002) Ultrasonographic evaluation of vertebral venous valves. AJNR Am J Neuroradiol 23(8):1418–1420

Part II
Intracranial veins

5 Ultrasound Machine: The Significance of Venous Preset

A reliable and dedicated setting of the ultrasound machine becomes crucial also for the study of the intracranial veins with transcranial color-coded duplex sonography (TCCS). It is necessary to start from what is known of the arterial district and to modify the individual parameters on the basis of the peculiar characteristics of the intracranial venous circulation, which is, however, characterized by the lack of valves. Therefore, the flow direction in each vein and sinus is directly driven by the pressure gradient and by the flow velocity, which is definitely lower than the one of the arteries.

A sectorial phased array probe is employed, with the emission frequency ranging between 1.5 and 2.5 MHz for adults. A frequency of between 1.5 and 2.0 MHz usually represents the best compromise between the attenuation caused by the skull bone and the need to reach a depth of 14–15 cm both for the B-mode and for the color mode or power mode. Both modes can be used in studying the cerebral veins. Although the first allows to evaluate directly the flow direction in the vessel, the second permits to have a more favorable signal/noise ratio. Besides, with appropriate persistence controlling, the color/power mode assures a more stable image under the dynamic conditions due to the venous examination.

In fact, due to the low flow velocity in the cerebral veins, it is first necessary to minimize or even reset the low-pass filter of the incoming signal, so as not to cut a portion of the venous flows. Besides, in order to reduce the PRF (up to 0.5 kHz or lower) as much as possible, the gain needs to be gradually increased up to the limit of the noise. The excessive reduction in the PRF, although necessary, can make the background noise and the artifact component even more evident, since the latter is related to the vibration and the intracranial structures pulsatility on account of the consequent frame rate reduction. These drawbacks can often be avoided by using the power mode [1].

Electronic supplementary material Supplementary material is available in the online version of this chapter at http://dx.doi.org/10.1007/978-88-470-5465-3_5. Videos can also be accessed at http://www.springerimages.com/videos/978-88-470-5465-3

G. Malferrari et al., *Neurosonological Evaluation of Cerebral Venous Outflow*,
DOI: 10.1007/978-88-470-5465-3_5, © Springer-Verlag Italia 2014

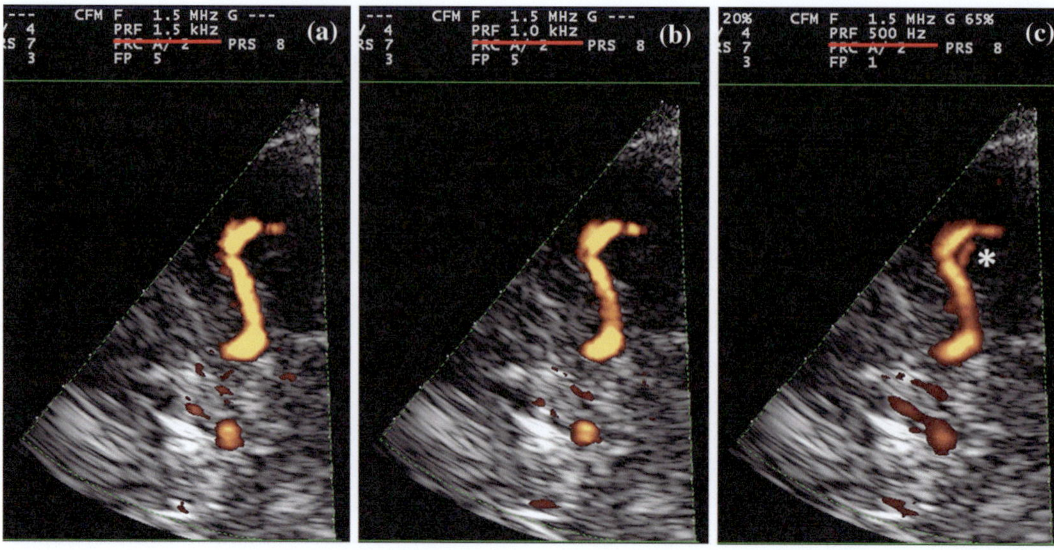

Fig. 5.1 **a–c** The picture shows an example of the effect of decreasing PRF in the ultrasound preset for venous study in power mode. TCCS from the temporal bone window in axial scanning plane, focused on middle cerebral artery (MCA) and deep middle cerebral vein (dMCV) in power mode, using progressively reduced PRF values from **a** to **c**. While MCA seems always easily identifiable, also with PRF values of 1.5 kHz (**a**), the power signal corresponding to the dMCV does not appear until the PRF value decreases to 0.5 kHz (**c**) (*asterisk*)

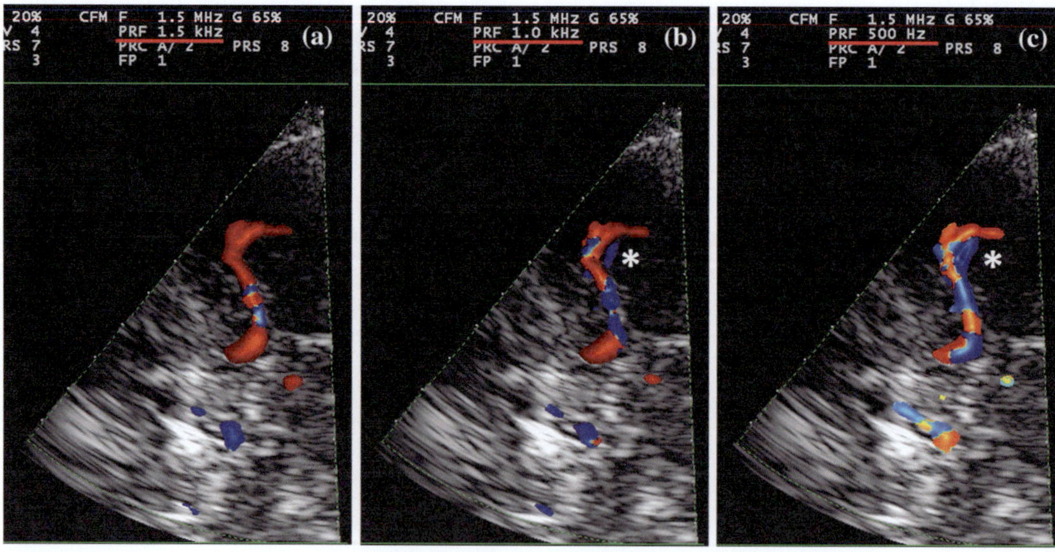

Fig. 5.2 **a–c** The picture shows an example of the effect of decreasing PRF in the ultrasound preset for venous study in color mode. TCCS from the temporal bone window in axial scanning plane, focused on MCA and dMCV in color mode, using progressively reduced PRF values from a to c. While MCA seems always easily identifiable, also with PRF values of 1.5 kHz (**a**), the color signal corresponding to the dMCV appears at PRF values of 1.0 kHz (**b**) (*asterisk*) and it is more evident at the PRF value of 0.5 kHz (**c**) (*asterisk*)

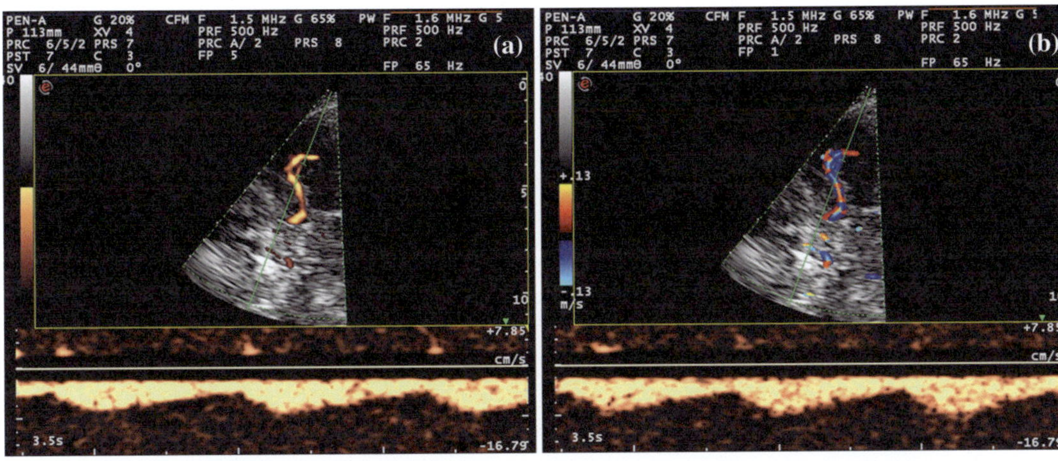

Fig. 5.3 **a**, **b** For a further confirmation of the vascular nature of the structure signaled in power mode and in color mode in the previous figure as the dMCV, the Doppler waveform is sampled at the level of the M1-M2 MCA passage and its morphology is congruent with a venous vessel with a flow direction away from the probe, as the dMCV at its insular end, either in power mode (**a**) and in color mode (**b**)

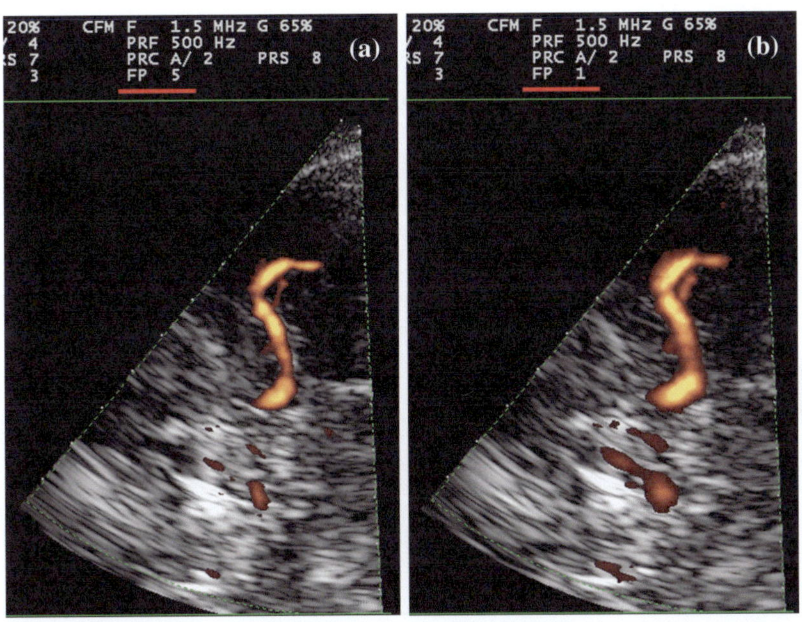

Fig. 5.4 TCCS from the temporal bone window in axial scanning plane in power mode, focusing on dMCV. The decrease in wall filter allows a full identification of the vessels, particularly veins (*right* part of the figure in comparison with the *left* one)

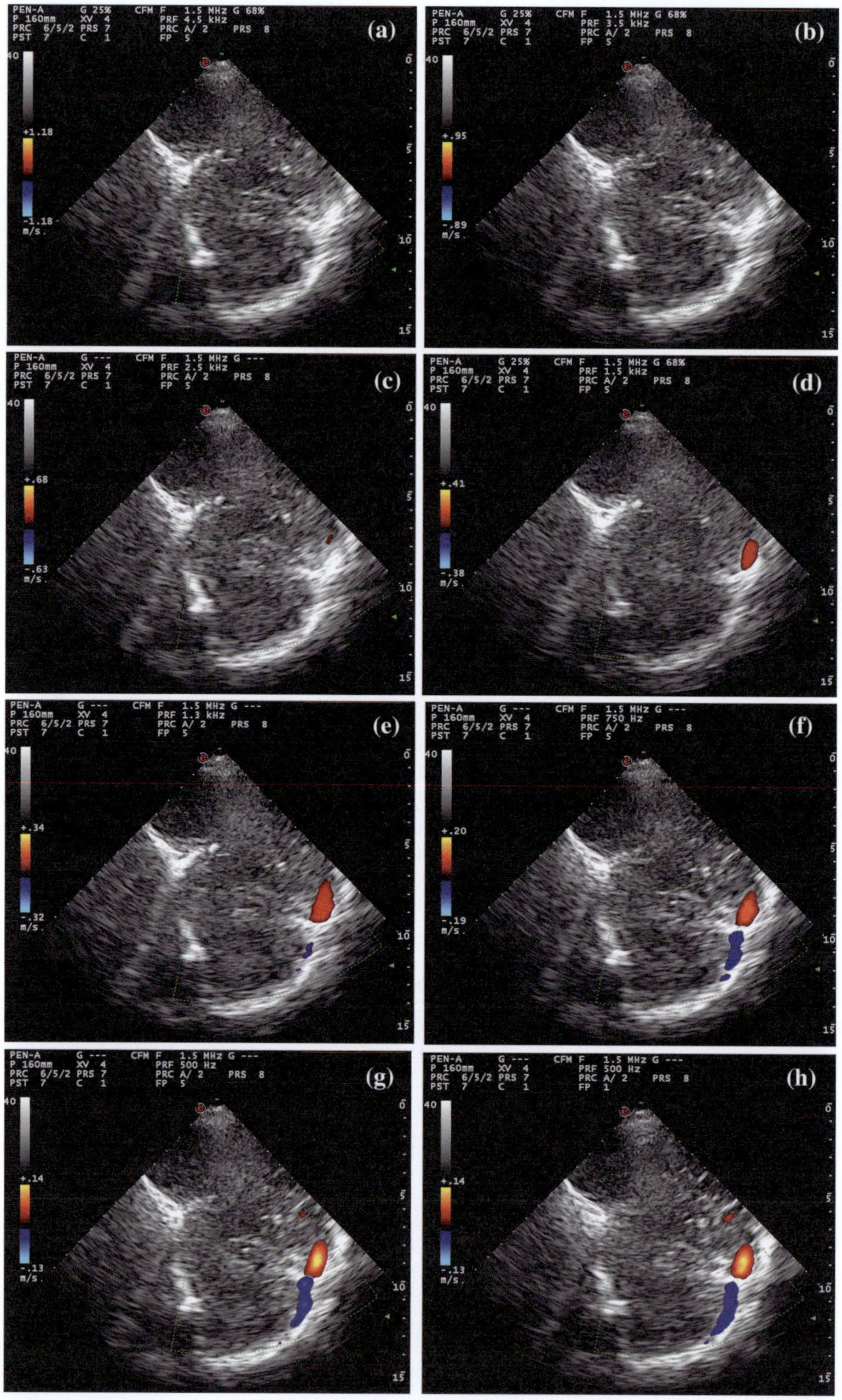
(a)
(b)
(c)
(d)
(e)
(f)
(g)
(h)

◀ **Fig. 5.5** **a–h** TCCS from temporal bone window in axial scanning plane in color mode, with approach for posterior cranial fossa and *color box* pointed on the ipsilateral and contralateral TS. It can be seen in the series of pictures from **a** to **g** a progressively decreasing PRF value of color mode from 4.5 to 0.5 kHz with the first appearance of the color signal of the ipsilateral TS (starting from picture **c** at PRF 2.5 kHz), which becomes more and more evident decreasing the PRF until to see also the contralateral TS in picture **e** (PRF 1.3 kHz). A subsequent decrease in PRF makes possible to better see the course of the contralateral TS until a PRF value of 0.5 kHz (picture **g**). In picture **h**, there is the same scan as in picture **g** but without wall filter, producing a further increase in the flow signal that can be received and imaged

Reference

1. Malferrari G, Zedde M (2012) Guida pratica allo studio sonologico del distretto venoso extra ed intracranico. Edizioni La Dotta

Ultrasound Anatomy and How to do the Examination

6

6.1 Anatomical Remarks

The venous drainage of the cerebral hemispheres is carried out through two systems: the superficial venous system and the deep venous system [1–4].

The first one drains the cortex and the white matter surface through the cortical veins, with subsequent confluence into the dural sinuses. Among these, two important structures are the superior sagittal sinus (SSS), which drains the dorsolateral regions, and the CS, which drains the anterior and ventral region. The SSS begins at the foramen cecum and runs along the curvature of the internal surface of the skull, inside the dura mater layers, till it reaches the confluence of the sinuses, the torcular Herophili, and subsequently drains into the TS. It flows symmetrically from both sides in only 20 % of cases and in an asymmetrical manner in more than 50 %, based on the configuration of the torcular Herophili [1–4].

In 20 % of cases, the TS of one side completely drains the SSS (most often the right) and the one of the other side drains the straight sinus (SRS) who belongs to the deep venous system [4]. The CS extends from the superior orbital fissure to the apex of the petrous bone. It drains the orbital region and the middle cranial fossa. From the CS, the blood drains posterolaterally along the superior petrosal sinus (SPS) into the TS and the infero-laterally along the IPS into the SyS.

On the other hand, the deep venous system drains the deep white matter, the regions surrounding the lateral ventricles, and the third ventricle or basal cisterns [1–14]. The choroidal vein, the septal vein, and the thalamostriate vein unite just below the interventricular Monro's foramen to originate the internal cerebral vein (ICV), a paired structure, which runs in the roof of the third ventricle, and subsequently in the splenium of the corpus callosum, joins with the basal vein of Rosenthal (BVR) and the homologous contralateral one to form the Galen vein (GV), unpaired and in the midline.

The GV is a short and thin vein (1–2 cm long) which passes postero-superiorly next to the splenium of the corpus callosum into the quadrigeminal cistern. The ICV and the GV receive the BVR and the veins of the posterior fossa and drain in the anterior head of the SRS, at its union with the inferior sagittal sinus (ISS). The BVR begins at the anterior perforated substance by the union of the anterior cerebral vein, the dMCV, and the striated vein. The BVR of each side surrounds the midbrain with an orientation both inferior-superior and anterior-posterior to join the GV [5, 6]. The main collector of the deep venous system is the SRS, which receives the venous blood from the GV and flows into the TS, sometimes bilaterally, but more often with preferential discharge in the left

Electronic supplementary material Supplementary material is available in the online version of this chapter at http://dx.doi.org/10.1007/978-88-470-5465-3_6. Videos can also be accessed at http://www.springerimages.com/videos/978-88-470-5465-3

G. Malferrari et al., *Neurosonological Evaluation of Cerebral Venous Outflow*,
DOI: 10.1007/978-88-470-5465-3_6, © Springer-Verlag Italia 2014

TS [4]. The BVR is an important collateral route of the ICV and the GV and is substantially constant. In 5 % of cases, its post-peduncular tract is essentially hypoplastic, preferentially draining the system of the CS via the lateral mesencephalic vein [6].

The venous drainage of the posterior cranial fossa depends on the Galenic and petrosal system and, to a lesser degree, from the tentorial veins and TS [1–3].

6.2 Ultrasound Examination

The neurosonological study of the cerebral venous structures through TCCS has been well established in the last 20 years. The approaches and scanning planes for the major veins and venous sinuses which can be visualized with ultrasound have been well defined [8, 9, 15]. The technological developments still leave space to the development and validation of study approaches that allow to view different segments of the same structures or to increase the rate of insonation of some veins and sinuses as compared to the already defined methodologies. This development exploits the possibility to use multiple levels of insonation for the venous system study, based on the ultrasound anatomy knowledge and the development of a three-dimensional map of intracranial vascular structures and their anatomical relationships.

The examination usually begins from the temporal window with an axial access, in mesencephalic plane, similarly to the arterial study, and then goes on standardized planes according to the venous structure that needs to be studied. With the setting adjustments described in the previous chapter, this first approach allows to view the dMCV. It begins with the MCA, and it is more easily identifiable in correspondence of the passage between the M1 and M2 segments of the MCA. Its flow direction is away from the transducer. Pointing the probe downwards, through a slow inclination, it is possible to move, by means of a pontine plane, toward the bony structures of the middle cranial fossa, and then in the direction of the outflow region of the CS. At the same time, it is possible to identify the sphenoparietal sinus (SPaS), using as landmarks the edge of the small wing of the sphenoid bone and the medial head of the SPS, near the pyramid of the sphenoid bone, at the extreme medial edge of the petrous bone. Both sinuses present a flow direction that is away from the probe.

On the other hand, tilting the probe in the opposite direction, from mesencephalic to diencephalic plane, it is possible to view the BVR. This vein has the same course as the posterior cerebral artery (PCA), both in the pre-peduncular segment, with the flow direction approaching the probe, and in the post-peduncular segment, with the flow direction away from the probe and with the course slightly more cranial compared to the PCA. Also, the flow direction of the BVR segments coincides with the one of the corresponding PCA segments.

Following the more distal part of the BVR, on the diencephalic plane, it is possible to view the GV, which is placed posteriorly as to the hyperechoic signal of the pineal gland in the midline, with the flow direction away from the probe. With this scanning plane, the posterior head of the SSS can be simultaneously displayed, also with a direction away from the probe.

Table 6.1 Normal values of flow velocity of cerebral veins and sinuses [10–13]

	PSV (cm/sec)	EDV (cm/sec)	Detection rate (%)
TCCS, temporal bone window			
dMCV	4–15	3–11	53–95
BV	7–20	5–15	85–100
GCV	6–32	4–25	84–94
SRS	6–39	4–27	23–82
TS	6–56	5–38	20–84
SSS	6–20	3–14	36–67
SPaS	27 ± 17		84
SPS	27 ± 17		84
TCD, occipital window			
IPS	20 ± 9		78

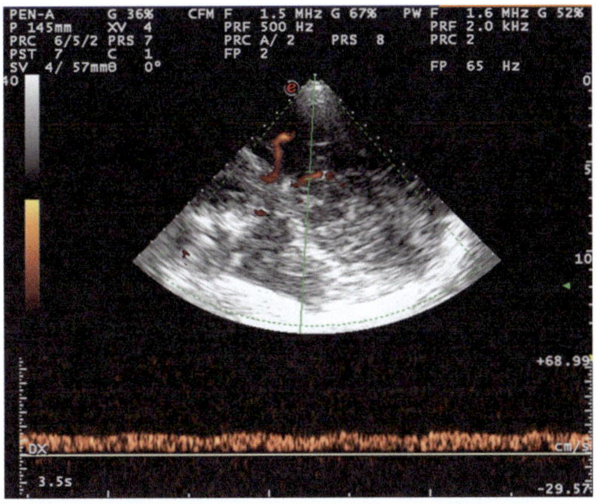

Fig. 6.1 Power-mode TCCS from temporal window in axial scanning plane (mesencephalic plane). The ipsilateral basal vein of Rosenthal is sampled in the prepeduncular segment, with flow direction toward the probe

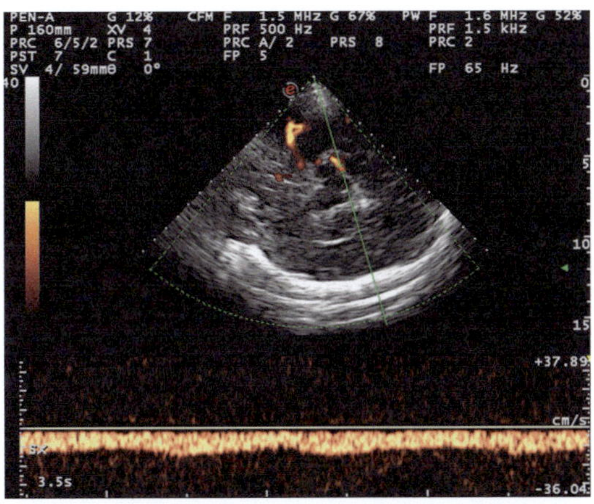

Fig. 6.2 TCCS from temporal window in axial scanning plane (diencephalic plane) in power mode. The ipsilateral BVR is sampled in the post-peduncular segment, with flow direction away from the probe, like the P3 PCA segment which was co-sampled

To continue from the GV to the SRS, which runs along the insertion of the tentorium on the falx, the scanning plane must be changed by tilting the probe postero-superiorly and slightly rotating a few degrees in the direction of the internal occipital protuberance, until the torcular Herophili or confluence of sinuses is reached. Also, the SRS has the flow direction away from the probe.

Another venous structure that can be visualized by ultrasounds is the TS; it can be insonated through a contralateral and ipsilateral approach. The latter one helps to increase the rate of global insonation and to view besides the proximal segment also the medium and distal ones of the TS, exploiting a more anterior window and using the bony landmark as a guide.

The classic contralateral approach, when the torcular Herophili has been visualized, requires a lower tilting of the probe until the proximal segment of the TS, adherent to the skull bone, can be seen; the flow direction is away from the probe.

The use of the occipital window is almost exclusively limited to the display of the IPS, at the side of the basilar artery with flow direction toward to the probe. It is possible to view, although with lower rates of insonation, also the SRS, the GV, and the ICV.

The main features of the intracranial veins flow waveform are represented by:

- Low flow velocity compared to the corresponding arteries;
- "Continuous" flow appearance throughout the cardiac cycle, maintaining, however, a pulsatility which at times becomes more evident;
- The need for an activation maneuver (Valsalva maneuver) to verify the nature of the venous flow in case of strong pulsatility.

Yet, the response to the Valsalva maneuver can vary in relation to the outflow activated, to the anatomical and functional variability, to the pressure gradient in a system with no valves, as well as to the influence of the continence of the IJV valve.

The normal values of the of venous flow velocity for the main intracranial vessels in healthy subjects have been defined in different studies and are shown in Table 6.1 [8].

Although the rate of identification of few veins and sinuses is generally quite high, there are, however, some differences with fairly broad range, in particular as regards the posterior fossa veins. The inter-operator reproducibility and reliability are not dissimilar to those reported for the arterial system.

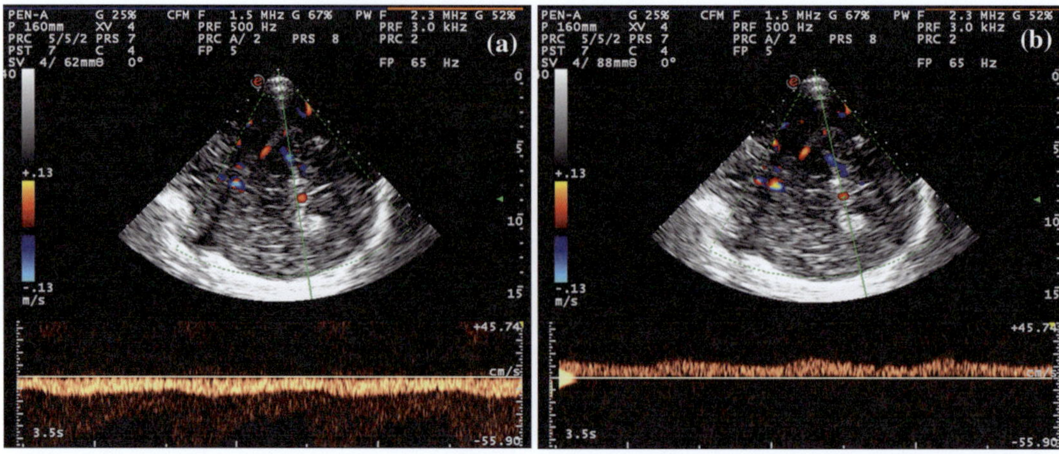

Fig. 6.3 **a**, **b** TCCS from temporal window in axial scanning plane (diencephalic plane) in color mode. In picture (**a**), the ipsilateral BVR is sampled in the post-peduncular segment, with flow direction away from the probe, like the P3 PCA segment, co-sampled. In picture (**b**), the contralateral post-peduncular BVR is sampled, with flow direction toward the probe as expected. The flow waveform shows an evident pulsatility; the systolic to diastolic range is lower compared to arterial waveform

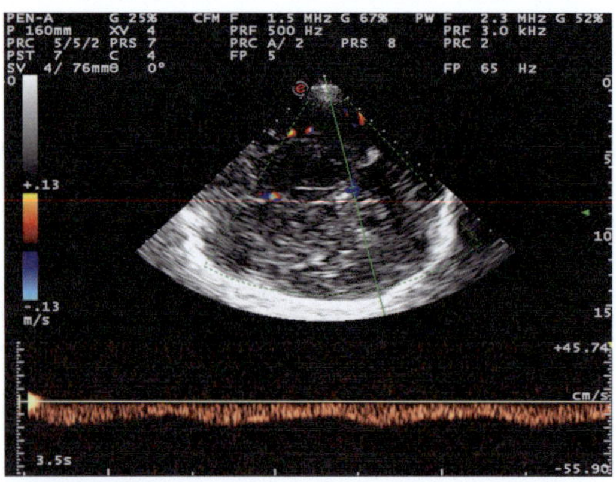

Fig. 6.4 TCCS from temporal widow in axial scanning plane (diencephalic plane) in color mode. Behind the hyperechoic image of the pineal gland, the GV is sampled, with flow direction away from the probe and a Doppler waveform similar to the previous one observed on the BVR

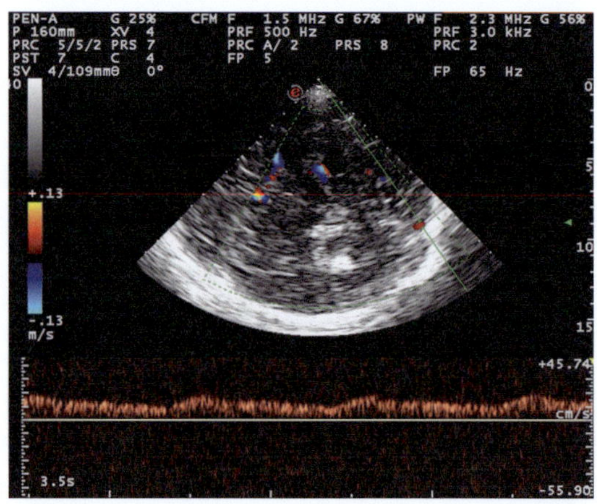

Fig. 6.5 TCCS from temporal window in axial scanning plane (low diencephalic plane) in color mode. The post-peduncular BVR (*yellow asterisk*) and the posterior segment of the SSS (*green asterisk*) are imaged. The SSS has a flow direction toward the probe and a Doppler waveform similar to the previous one of the BVR

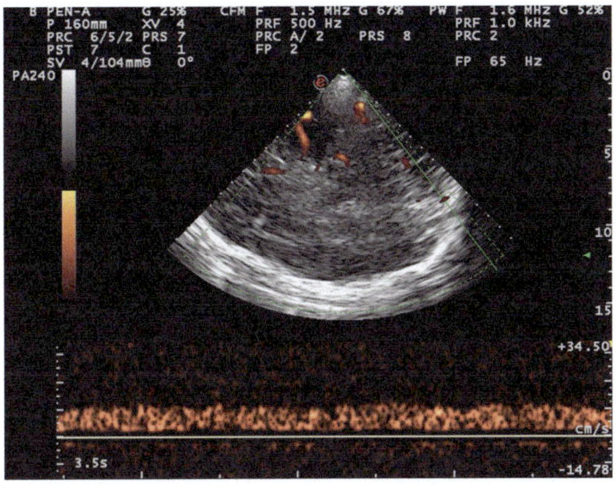

Fig. 6.6 TCCS from temporal window in axial scanning plane in power mode. The post-peduncular BVR (*yellow asterisk*) and the posterior segment of the SSS (*green asterisk*) are imaged. The SSS has a flow direction toward the probe and a Doppler waveform similar to the previous one of the BVR

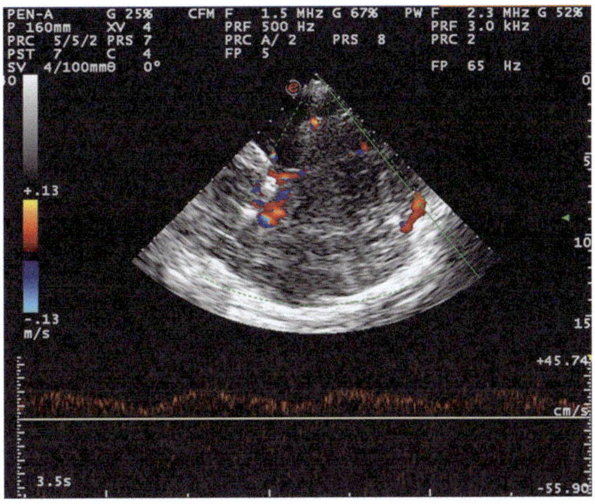

Fig. 6.7 TCCS from temporal widow in axial scanning plane in color mode; posterior cranial fossa approach for the insonation of the proximal segment of the ipsilateral TS, sampled near the confluens of sinuses. See the following detailed image for the parenchymal landmarks

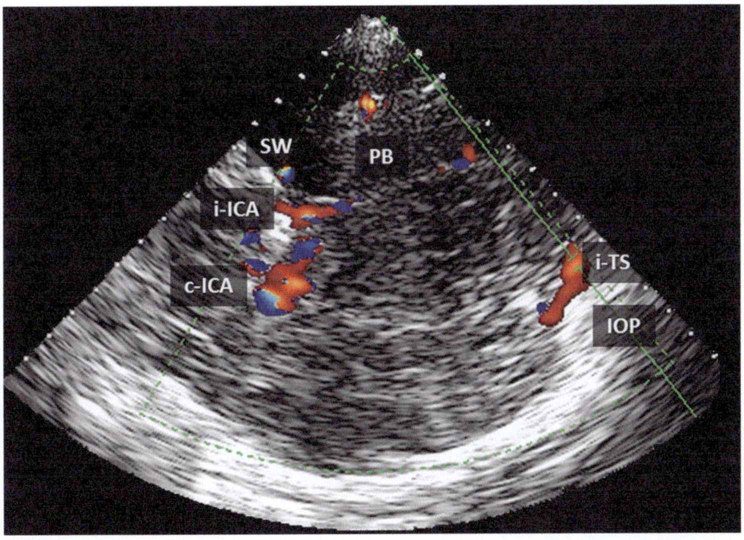

Fig. 6.8 TCCS from temporal window in axial scanning plane in color mode; posterior cranial fossa approach for the insonation of the proximal segment of the ipsilateral TS. The following structures are imaged: i-ICA ipsilateral internal carotid artery. C-ICA contralateral internal carotid artery. IOP internal occipital protuberance. PB edge of the ipsilateral petrous bone. SW edge of the ipsilateral sphenoid wing. i-TS ipsilateral transverse sinus

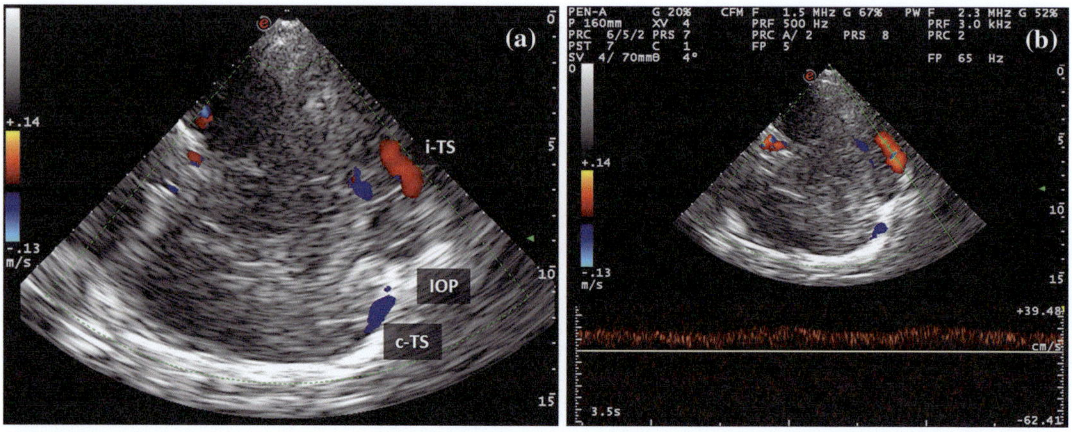

Fig. 6.9 **a**, **b** TCCS from temporal window in axial scanning plane in color mode. This is an extreme approach for insonating the middle segment of the ipsilateral TS (*red arrow*) (picture **a**), whose Doppler waveform is imaged in picture (**b**)

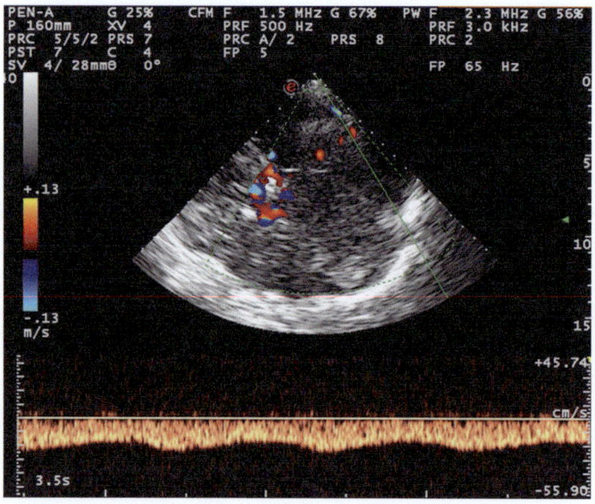

Fig. 6.10 TCCS from temporal window in axial scanning plane in color mode; posterior cranial fossa approach for the insonation of the distal segment of the ipsilateral TS, sampled near the confluence of the superior petrous sinus (SPS). The insonation plane is slightly more angled than the plane used for the insonation of the proximal segment of the ipsilateral TS, and the approach is in an oblique pontine plane. See the following detailed image for the parenchymal landmarks

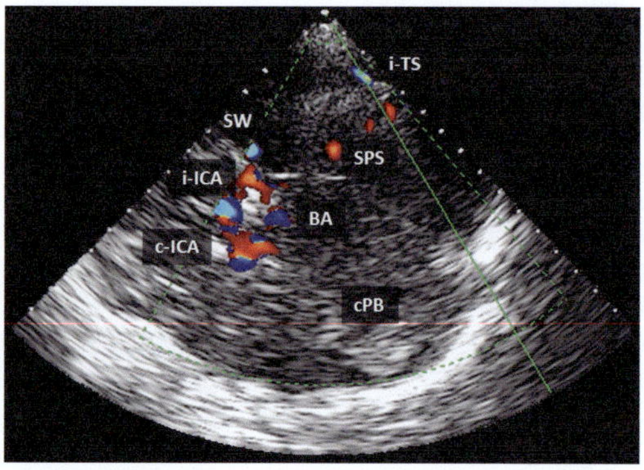

Fig. 6.11 TCCS from temporal window in axial scanning plane in color mode; posterior cranial fossa approach for the insonation of the distal segment of the ipsilateral TS. The following structures are imaged: i-ICA Ipsilateral internal carotid artery. C-ICA contralateral internal carotid artery. BA basilar artery. cPB edge of the contralateral petrous bone. SW edge of the ipsilateral sphenoid wing. SPS superior petrous sinus. i-TS ipsilateral transverse sinus

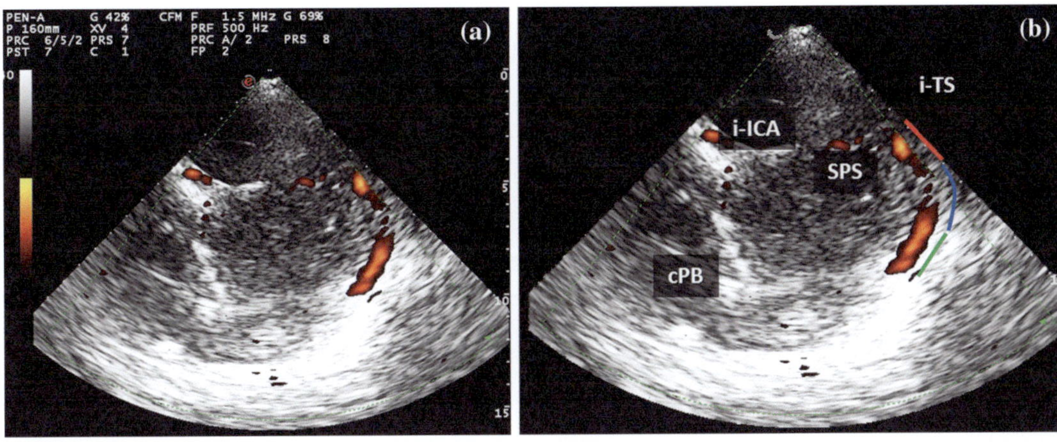

Fig. 6.12 TCCS from temporal window in axial scanning plane in power mode; extreme posterior cranial fossa approach for the insonation of the ipsilateral TS. The following structures are imaged: i-ICA Ipsilateral internal carotid artery. cPB edge of the contralateral petrous bone. SPS superior petrous sinus. i-TS ipsilateral transverse sinus. The ipsilateral transverse sinus is imaged along its entire course, allowing to distinguish: (1) proximal segment, (2) middle segment, (3) distal segment

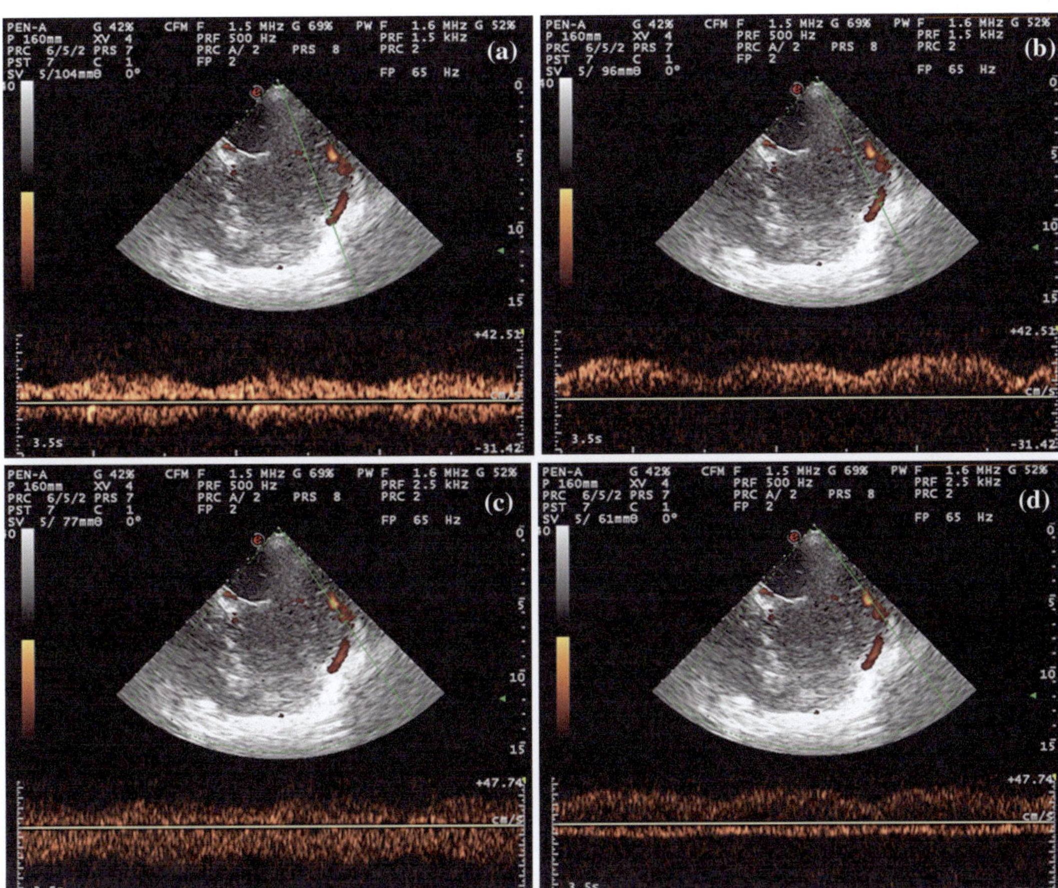

Fig. 6.13 TCCS from temporal window in axial scanning plane in power mode; extreme posterior cranial fossa approach for the insonation of the ipsilateral TS. From *top* to *bottom*, the following segments are sampled with Doppler signal. **a** Confluens of sinuses with bidirectional flow. **b** Proximal segment of TS, with a flow directed toward the probe. **c** A middle segment with a bidirectional flow and a curved course. **d** A distal segment with a clearer flow directed away from the probe

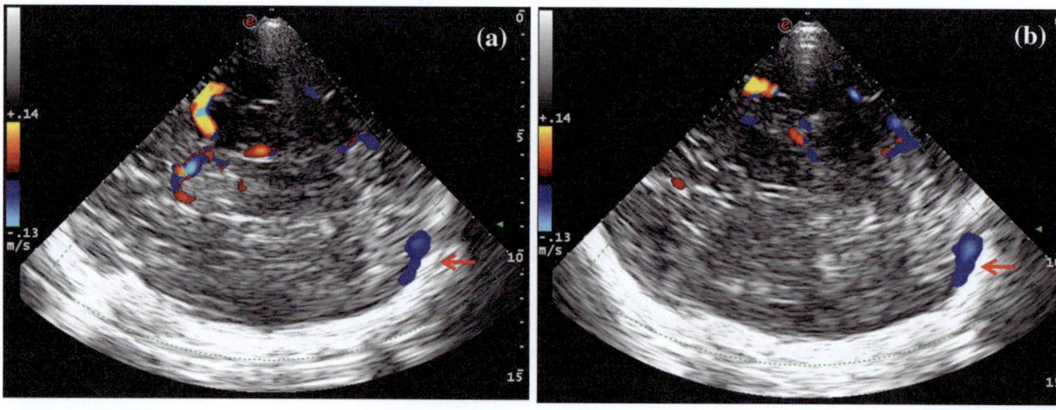

Fig. 6.14 **a**, **b** TCCS from temporal window in axial scanning plane in color mode. The picture illustrates the most used approach for insonating the contralateral TS, starting from a mesencephalic plane with the anterior visualization of M1 MCA course up to the M1–M2 passage and the posterior appearance of the color-coded signal of the contralateral TS along the skull (picture **a**). The posterior persistence of the contralateral TS (picture **b**) can be displayed by means of a slight tilting of the probe to the diencephalic approach in order to visualize M2 MCA anteriorly. The TS is indicated by the *red arrow*. In the following figures, parenchymal landmarks are more detailed

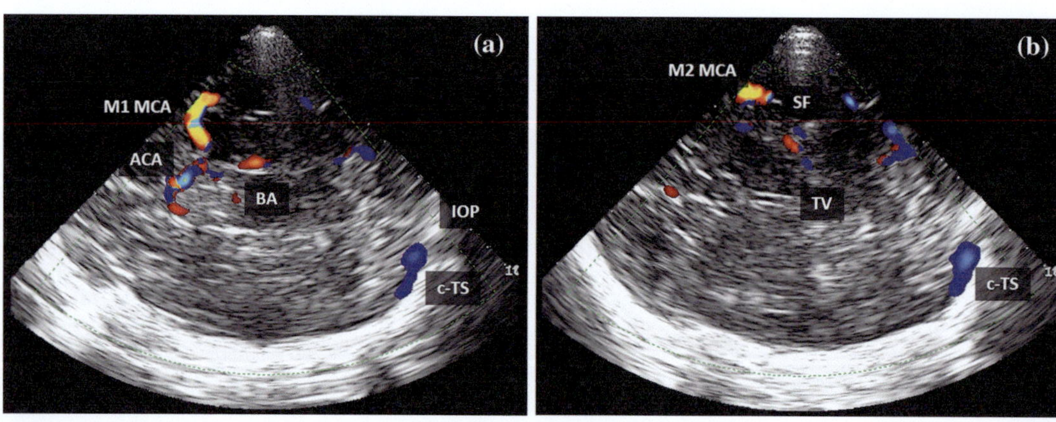

Fig. 6.15 TCCS from temporal window in axial scanning plane in color mode. The figure above shows the mesencephalic plane and the figure below the diencephalic plane. The parenchymal landmarks and vessels are as follows: M1 MCA ipsilateral MCA in the M1 segment. M2 MCA ipsilateral MCA in the M2 segment. ACA ipsilateral A1 anterior cerebral artery. SF sylvian fissure. IOP internal occipital protuberance. c-TS contralateral transverse sinus. TV third ventricle. BA basilar artery

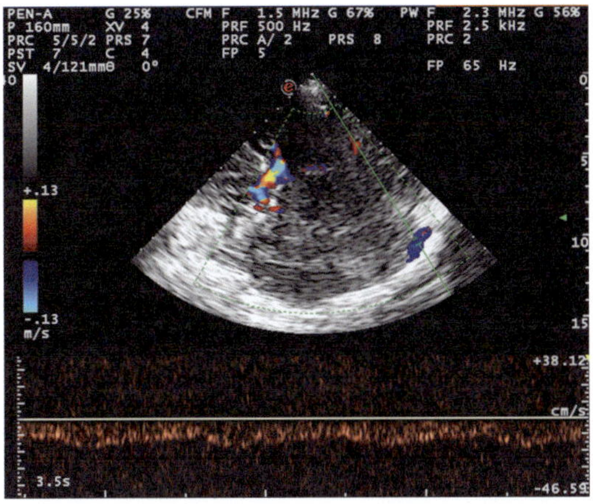

Fig. 6.16 TCCS from temporal window in axial scanning plane in color mode; posterior cranial fossa approach for the insonation of the proximal segment of the ipsilateral TS, sampled near the confluens of sinuses. See the following detailed image for the parenchymal landmarks

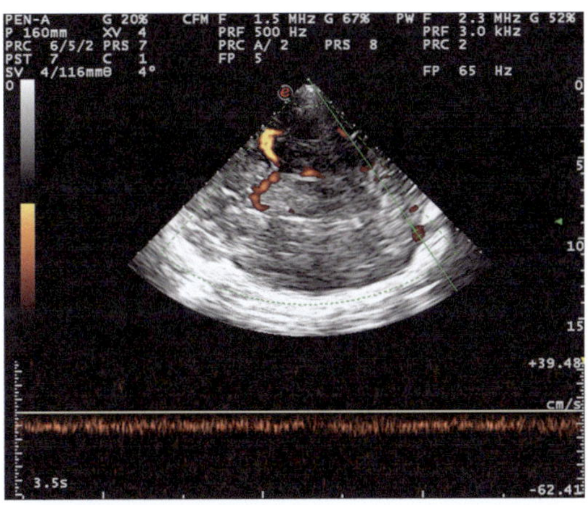

Fig. 6.17 TCCS from temporal window in axial scanning plane in power mode. The contralateral TS is insonated in a modified mesencephalic plane, corresponding to the one illustrated in Fig. 6.14 in color mode. The TS is indicated by the red arrow, and the Doppler waveform shows a continuous trace with a very low pulsatility

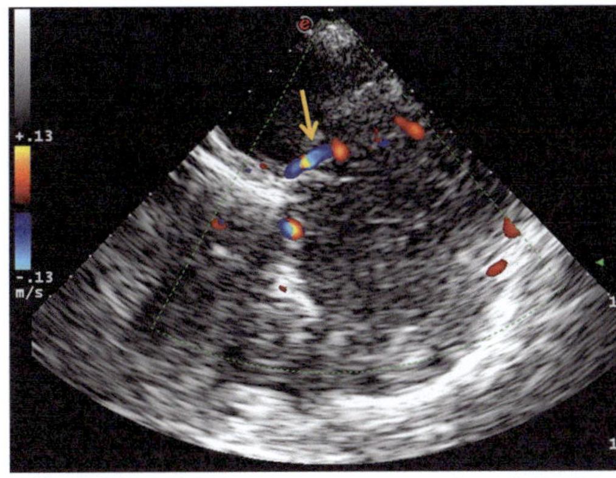

Fig. 6.18 TCCS from temporal window in axial scanning plane in color mode; posterior cranial fossa approach for the insonation of the medial head of the SPS. The insonation plane is oriented toward the basicranium and to the posterior cranial fossa. The ipsilateral SPS is indicated by the *yellow arrow*. The flow direction of the medial head of the SPS is usually away from the probe; in the other segment, it is possible to see a flow direction toward the probe (see Figs. 6.21, 6.22). See the following detailed image for the parenchymal landmarks

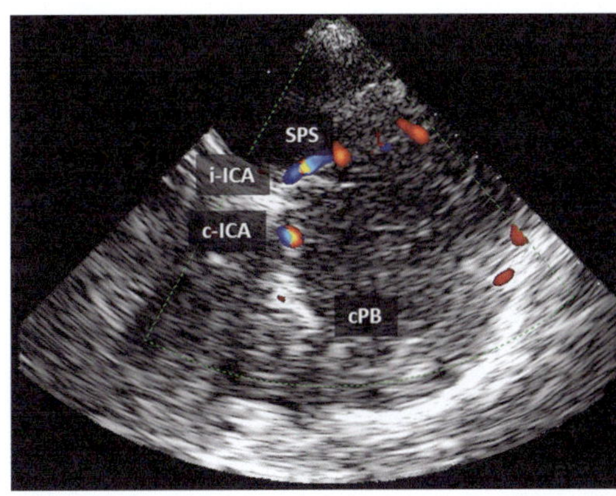

Fig. 6.19 TCCS from temporal window in axial scanning plane in color mode; posterior cranial fossa approach for the insonation of the medial head of the SPS. The following structures are imaged: i-ICA Ipsilateral internal carotid artery. C-ICA contralateral internal carotid artery. cPB edge of the contralateral petrous bone. SPS superior petrous sinus

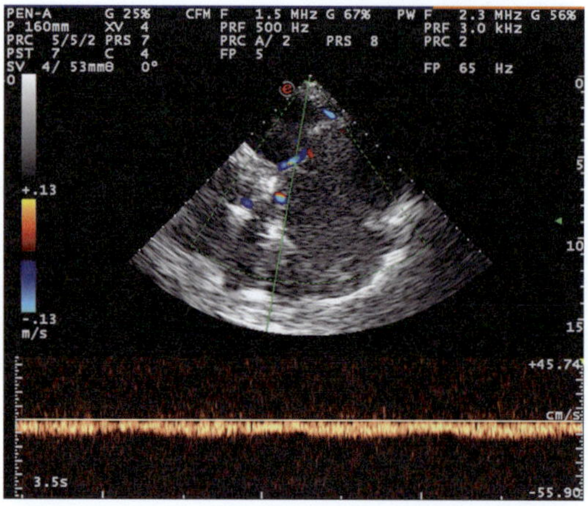

Fig. 6.20 TCCS from temporal window in axial scanning plane in color mode; posterior cranial fossa approach for the insonation of the medial head of the SPS. The Doppler waveform of the SPS shows a flow direction away from the probe and a low pulsatility index

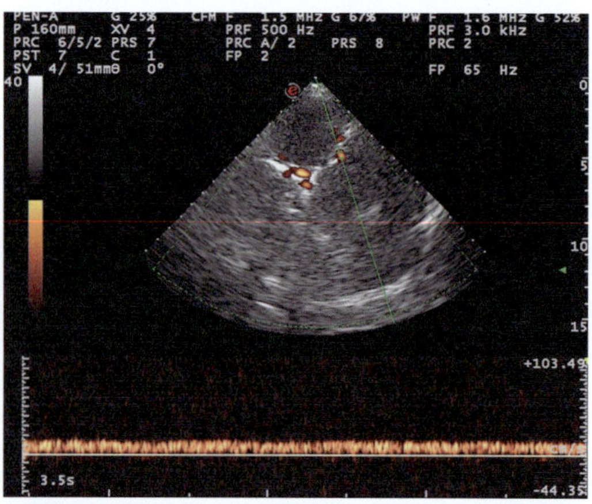

Fig. 6.21 TCCS from temporal window in axial scanning plane in color mode; posterior cranial fossa approach for the insonation of the medial head of the SPS. The Doppler waveform of the SPS shows a flow direction away from the probe and a low pulsatility index

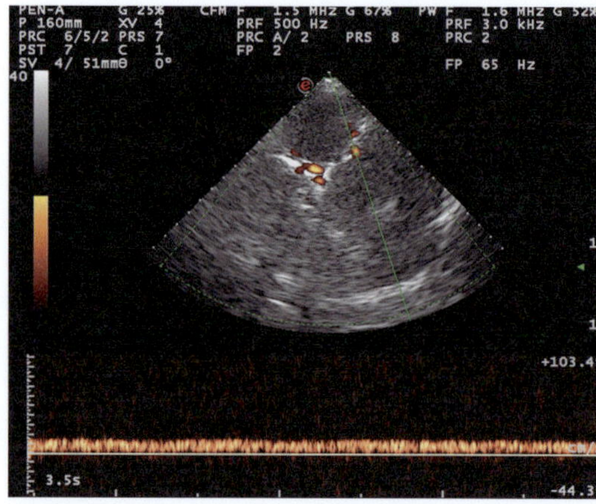

Fig. 6.22 Another example of the same segment of the SPS is obtained by using a different tilting of the probe

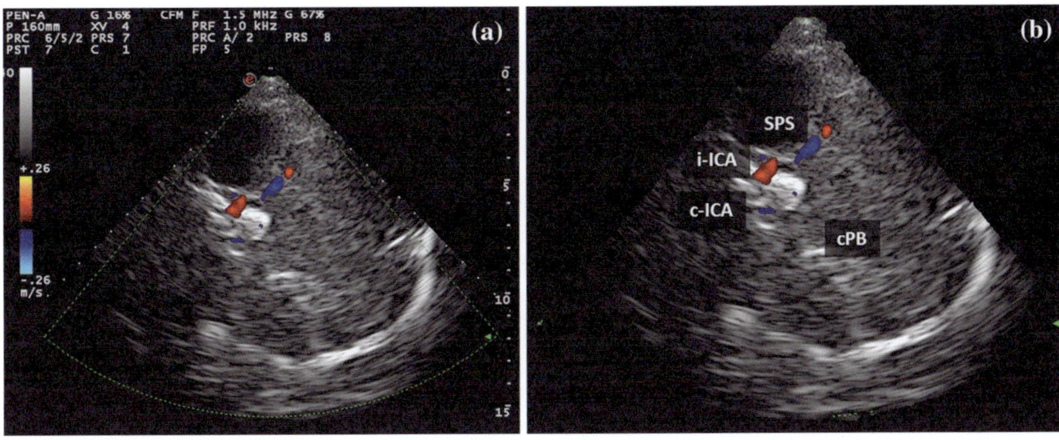

Fig. 6.23 **a**, **b** TCCS from temporal window in axial scanning plane in color mode; posterior cranial fossa approach for the insonation of the medial head of the SPS (picture **a**). The following structures are imaged (labeled in picture **b**): i-ICA Ipsilateral internal carotid artery. C-ICA contralateral internal carotid artery. cPB edge of the contralateral petrous bone. SPS superior petrous sinus

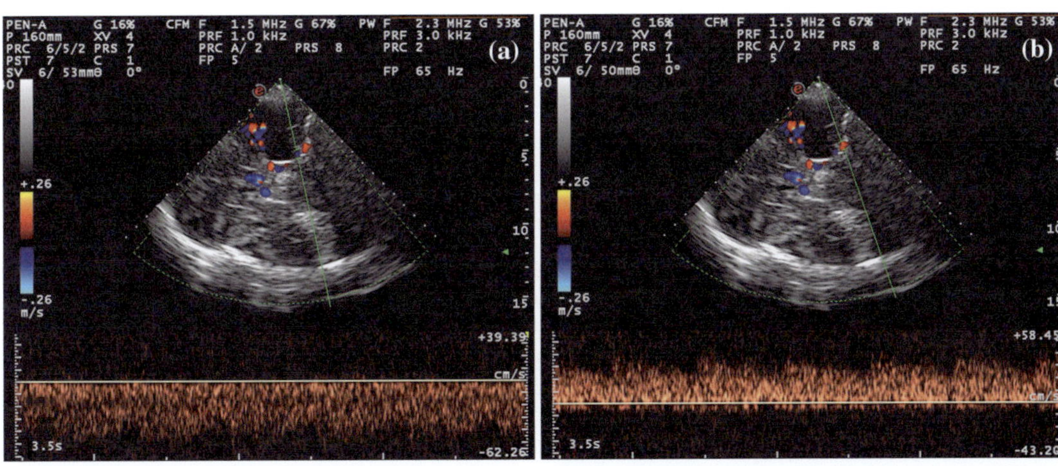

Fig. 6.24 **a**, **b** TCCS from temporal window in axial scanning plane in color mode, similar to the previous figures but with a slightly different tilting of the probe, so that the MCA is detectable. The Doppler waveform shows the different flow direction of contiguous segments of SPS, as previously inferred by the respective color-coded flow directions, away from the probe in picture (**a**) and toward the probe in picture (**b**)

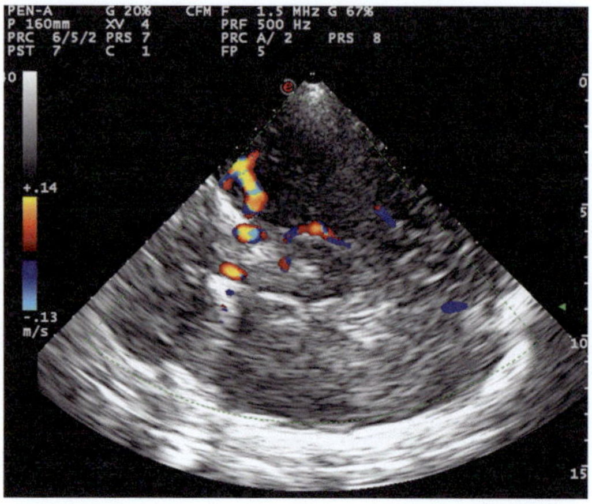

Fig. 6.25 TCCS from temporal window in axial scanning plane in color mode; oblique mesencephalic insonation plane for the SRS. The probe is tilted with the anterior tip oriented slightly above the posterior tip. In the *right* half of the image, in the midline, the color and flow signal of the SRS is visible along the hyperechoic insertion line of the cerebral falx on the cerebellar tentorium. The flow direction is away from the probe

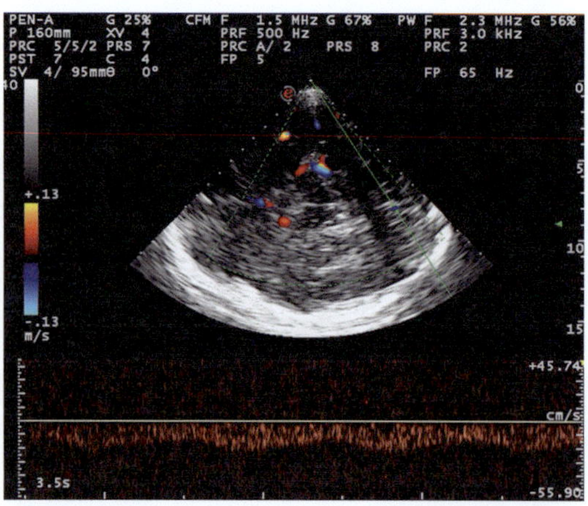

Fig. 6.26 TCCS from temporal window in axial scanning plane in color mode; oblique mesencephalic insonation plane for the straight sinus. The flow is sampled in the *midline* with a flow direction away from the probe and a Doppler waveform with the classic low pulsatility

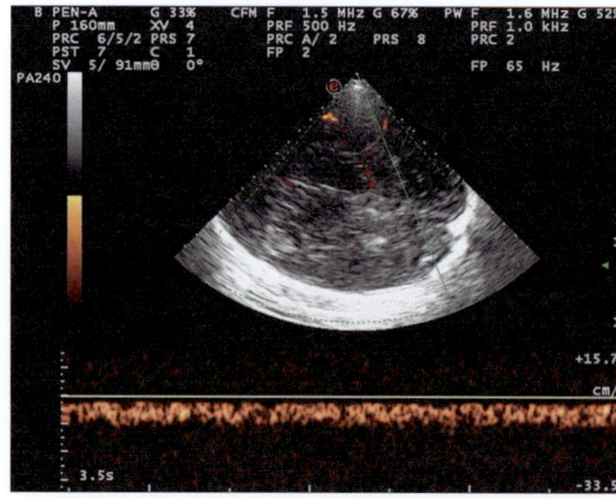

Fig. 6.27 TCCS from temporal window in axial scanning plane in power mode; diencephalic plane. With the probe tilting opposite to the one used in Fig. 6.26, the medial head of the SRS is imaged, showing a flow direction away from the probe

References

1. Schaller B (2004) Physiology of cerebral venous blood flow: from experimental data in animals to normal function in humans. Brain Res Brain Res Rev 46:243–260
2. Meder JF, Chiras J, Roland J et al (1994) Venous territories of the brain. J Neuroradiol 21:118–133
3. Schmidek HH, Auer LM, Kapp JP (1985) The cerebral venous system. Neurosurgery 17:663–678
4. Suzuki Y, Ikeda H, Shimadu M et al (2001) Variations of the basal vein: identification using three-dimensional CT angiography. AJNR Am J Neuroradiol 22:670–676
5. Taveras JM (1996) Angiography in neuroradiology, 3rd edn. Williams & Wilkins, Baltimore, p 998
6. Wolf BS, Newman CM, Schlesinger B (1955) The diagnostic value of the deep cerebral veins in cerebral angiography. Radiology 64:161–167
7. Ono M, Rhoton AL Jr, Peace D et al (1984) Microsurgical anatomy of the deep venous system of the brain. Neurosurgery 15:621–657
8. Erwin P (2008) Stolz, role of ultrasound in diagnosis and management of cerebral vein and sinus thrombosis. In: da Caso V, Agnelli G, Paciaroni M (eds) Handbook on cerebral venous thrombosis. Front neurol neuroscience Basel, Karger, vol 23, pp 112–121
9. Malferrari G. (Ed), Eco color doppler transcranico, Mattioli Editore 2007
10. Valdueza JM, Hoffmann O, Doepp F, Lehmann R, Einhäupl KM (1998) Venous Doppler ultrasound assessment of parasellar region. Cerebrovasc Dis 8:113–117
11. Stolz E, Kaps M, Kern A, Dorndorf W (1999) Frontal bone windows for transcranial color-coded duplex sonography. Stroke 30:814–820
12. Stolz E, Kaps M, Kern A, Babacan SS, Dorndorf W (1999) Transcranial color-coded duplex sonography of intracranial veins and sinuses in adults. Reference data from 130 volunteers. Stroke 30:1070–1075

13. Doepp F, Hoffmann O, Lehmann R, Einhaupl KM, Valdueza JM (1999) The inferior petrosal sinus: assessment by transcranial Doppler ultrasound using the suboccipital approach. J Neuroimaging 9:193–197
14. Stolz E, Babacan SS, Bodeker RH, Gerriets T, Kaps M (2001) Interobserver and intraobserver reliability of venous transcranial color-coded flow velocity measurements. J Neuroimaging 11:385–392
15. Malferrari G, Zedde M (2012) Guida Pratica allo studio sonologico del distretto venoso extra ed intracranico, Edizioni La Dotta

Main Pathological Pictures with Ultrasound

7

7.1 Cerebral Vein Thrombosis

The ultrasound findings in a subject with cerebral venous thrombosis can be different according to the course of the disease over time, and therefore, also the role of neurosonological technique changes in the various stages. For both aspects, the acute phase and the follow-up can be distinguished.

The first findings in the literature pertaining to TransCranial Doppler (TCD) findings refer to the identification of high flow velocity, which was ascribed to the collateral circle activation [1]. However, basically there is general agreement on the fact that such a methodology should not be the first choice to establish or to rule out a cerebral venous thrombosis. In fact, there is the possibility of a false-negative exam in half of the cerebral venous thrombosis cases, on account of the variability of the insonation rate in the different vessels and of the non-predictable activation of the collateral circle in the large venous vessels.

The pathological findings described in the literature are divided into direct and indirect signs.

The only direct finding is the absence of Color-mode or Power-mode signals inside a dural sinus after injecting ultrasound contrast medium. However, ultrasound methodology cannot by itself differentiate complete thrombosis from aplasia as well as partial thrombosis from hypoplasia.

The indirect findings relate to the identification of the collateral circle activation, which may present itself with the following patterns [2]:

- Several veins already displayed with arterial preset, due to high flow velocity
- High venous flow velocity (greater than standard +2 standard deviations) of the normal values on the outflow vessels activated as collateral routes
- Inverted flow direction in a patent venous vessel, such as the flow toward the probe on the BVR on both sides in case of thrombosis of the SRS
- Inter-hemispherical differences in the mean blood velocity of paired veins equal to >50 %, which must be associated abnormally with on side high velocity. In fact, such a unilateral finding could be ascribed to individual physiological characteristics.

Anyhow, the collateral circle activation may vary considerably. Well-known false-positive results are represented by high flow velocity either on the SPS or on the SPaS in close proximity to the terminal part of the CS, due to their physiological diameter reduction.

In the follow-up of cerebral venous thrombosis, neurosonological methodology may help to monitor the venous recanalization in subjects who

Electronic supplementary material Supplementary material is available in the online version of this chapter at http://dx.doi.org/10.1007/978-88-470-5465-3_7. Videos can also be accessed at http://www.springerimages.com/videos/978-88-470-5465-3

G. Malferrari et al., *Neurosonological Evaluation of Cerebral Venous Outflow*,
DOI: 10.1007/978-88-470-5465-3_7, © Springer-Verlag Italia 2014

have already been studied by means of neuroradiological imaging. However, a neurosonological study, normal *ab initio* or a normalization of the same within 90 days, is associated with an excellent functional outcome (mRS 0-1) [3].

7.2 Traumatic Brain Injury and Intracranial Hypertension

The increase in intracranial pressure is caused by space-occupying lesions; they show an evolving phase corresponding to the onset of a cerebral edema with a known trend over time, as in ischemic vascular lesions or in traumatic brain injury (TBI). This condition typically produces venous hemodynamic modifications in the adaptive and intracranial volume reduction mechanisms. These hemodynamic venous modifications affect the blood flow velocity which is measurable on single vessels and are associated with the prognosis and the onset of cerebral damage, especially in TBI. Furthermore, the intracranial hypertension deriving from space-occupying lesions may cause a traction and a compression of the vessels alongside the dural membranes (e.g. falx or tentorium cerebri).

As reported by Stolz et al. [4] in a study on patients affected by ischemic hemispheric stroke, the compression of the BVR at the level of the mesencephalic cistern or the GV at the junction with the SRS may cause blood velocity variations that can be monitored with TCCS. For instance, as regards the BVR, an increase in the blood flow velocity on the injured side can initially be observed (within 24 h from the event). It is followed by a significant decrease within 5 days, associated with an increase in the midline shift and to transtentorial herniation. On the SRS, the trend of blood flow velocity appears to be opposite, with a U-shaped curve, with an initial reduction followed by an increase when the median line shift is about 1–1.5 cm. On the other hand, in the GV, the blood flow velocity increase has been observed to occur in a sudden way with a midline shift >1.5 cm. All these alterations have been detected as the expression of the intracranial hypertension in patients with negative outcome, but not in the survivors. As a consequence, such findings may also have prognostic meaning.

7.3 Artero-Venous Malformations and Fistulas

The identification of cerebral artero-venous malformations (AVM) with TCCS depends on their dimension, location, and hemodynamic blood flow changes. Using only the B-mode imaging, large AVMs which have diameter > 4 cm can be detected. They are structures in which hypoechoic areas alternate with patchy hyperechoic ones. Color mode (and Power mode) allows to add the velocity and hemodynamic information, directly displaying the main afferent arteries, the vein outflow and the nidus, that is the vascular convolutions of the malformation. Besides, the afferent arteries are characterized, like in the arterio-venous fistulas (FAV), by low resistance indexes and by normal or high velocities depending on the hemodynamics of the malformation itself. The draining veins may show an "arterialized" waveform morphology, i.e., with resistance indexes similar to the ones of the arterial district.

For example, the ultrasound evidence of the afferent arteries is possible in 71 % of the cases, with a significant limit regarding the parieto-occipital and superficial localization and for the posterior cranial fossa, as well as small-dimension malformations [5–9].

Therefore, a negative ultrasound examination with TCCS does not exclude the presence of an AVM.

Also the FAVs are characterized by low-resistance waveform of the afferent arteries, due to the abnormal communication between the arterial and the venous bed. This means high flow velocity, both systolic and end-diastolic one, and a reduced resistance index [8, 10, 11].

The high-flow fistulas, due to their great volume shunt, are more easily identifiable because they are the location of hemodynamic alterations both in the afferent arteries and in the drainage veins.

Also the draining veins and sinuses may show alterations in the Doppler waveform, that is, an increased inflow and higher velocity and pseudo-arterial flow pattern [12–14].

The examination of extracranial vessels may provide some information on the study of dural FAV by showing the decrease in the flow resistance indexes of the ECA. The carotid-cavernous fistula is a special kind of FAV. If it is of direct type, it can be displayed also through the orbital window both in Color mode, as a wide, mosaic-like aliasing image, and in Doppler waveform congruent with the color-coded signal.

On the other hand, both the direct and the indirect carotid-cavernous fistulas, or dural fistulas, can show an abnormal pattern on the drainage veins.

Musical murmurs or cry seagull signals can sometimes be identified at the level of the nidus, as well as an extremely marked turbulence in the flow waveform.

A dural FAV can be diagnosed by using TCCS if at least one of the following criteria is met:

- Identification of high flow velocity on the venous drainage vessels
- Identification of inverted venous flow direction or easy detection of sinuses generally not recognizable with TCCS, such as SyS, ISS, IPS, and SPS.

Any venous flow velocity greater than 50 cm/s should be considered pathological, and it indicates that a neuroradiological examination is necessary [15].

The drainage through the cortical veins cannot be adequately detected with TCCS.

As regards the carotid-cavernous fistulas, however, there are very few studies which have reported ultrasound criteria for a hemodynamic classification [13, 16, 17].

In Type A, there is a reduced resistance index on the ICA with a greater flow volume. In Type B, both resistance index and flow volume are normal on the ICAs as well as on the ECAs. In Type C and D, the resistance index of the ECA is reduced and the flow volume is normal.

Ultrasound examination may not succeed in identifying fistulas of small dimensions. Besides, it may not be able to tell apart Type B, C, and D exactly, despite combining the extracranial and the intracranial evaluation both through the temporal and the orbital window.

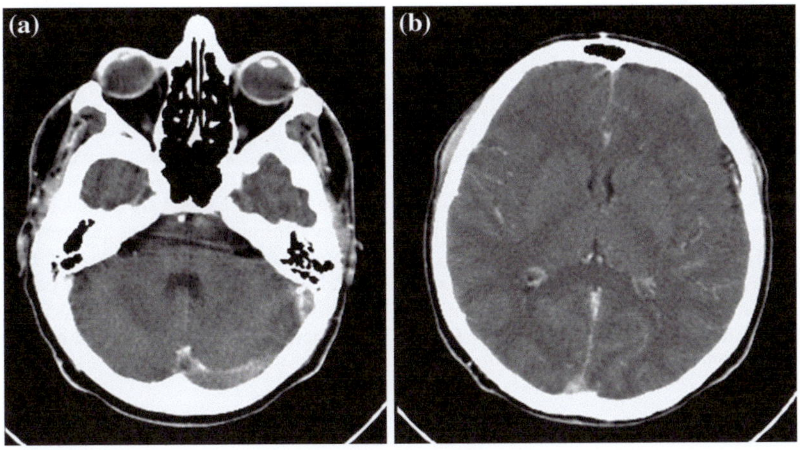

Fig. 7.1 Contrast-enhanced brain CT of a young patient with cerebral vein thrombosis, involving the *left* TS, the confluens of sinuses, and the distal end of the SSS. In the picture (**a**) is well evident the lack of endoluminal filling at the level of confluens of sinuses and *left* TS; in the picture (**b**) it can be seen the involvement of the posterior end of the SSS

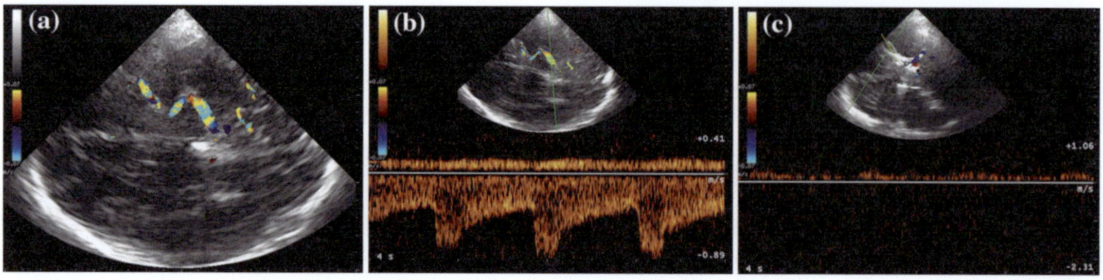

Fig. 7.2 **a–c** TCCS from temporal bone window in axial access (same subject of the previous figure). There are two of the indirect signs suggestive for the diagnosis of cerebral venous thrombosis, i.e., the presence of venous collateral vessels behind the diencephalon in the picture (**a**) and the inverted flow direction of a vein, i.e., *Right* BVR in the post-peduncular segment with flow direction to the probe, opposite to the direction of the P3 PCA simultaneously sampled (**b**). *Right* SPS with flow direction to the probe (**c**)

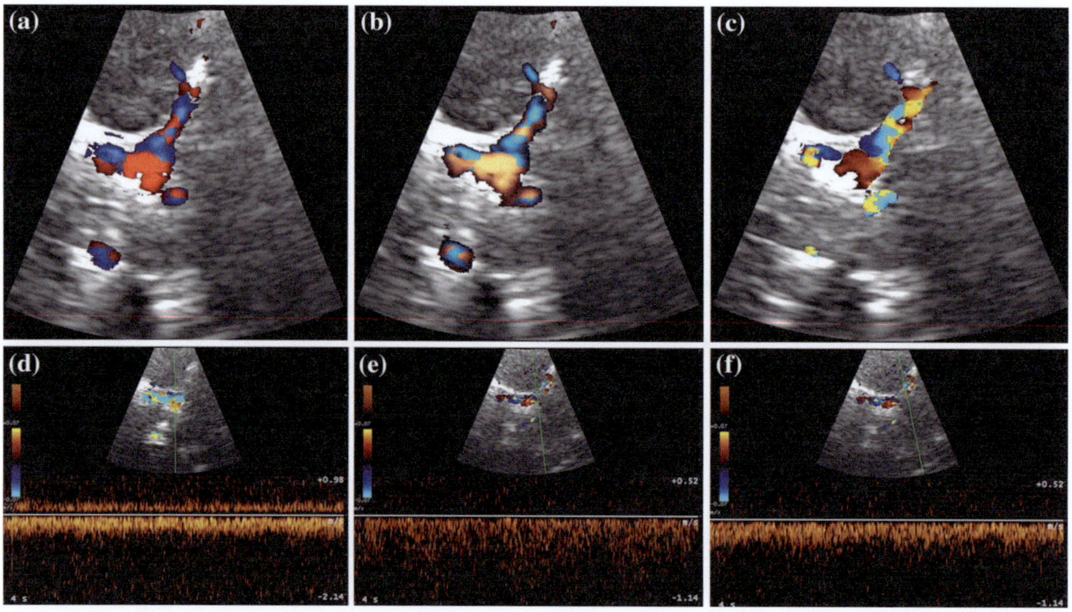

Fig. 7.3 **a–e** TCCS from the temporal bone window in axial scan (same subject of the previous figures). A further indirect sign of cerebral venous thrombosis can be seen, i.e., the increased flow velocity of a vein acting as alternative drainage route, as the SPS in this case. In the pictures (**a**) and (**b**), the medial end of the *left* SPS is insonated in Power mode with direction coding; in the picture (**c**), the same vein is insonated in Color mode with evident aliasing. In the pictures (**d–e**), the Doppler waveform is sampled in three sequential points of the medial segment of SPS, showing, particularly in picture (**e**), a markedly increased flow velocity with dispersion of frequencies in the waveform and orthograde direction

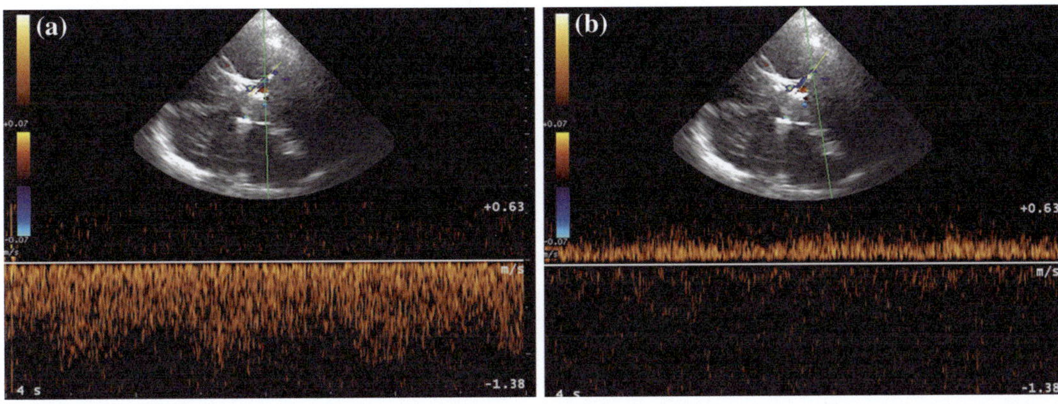

Fig. 7.4 **a** and **b** TCCS from temporal bone window in axial scan (same subjects of the previous figures). It shows another indirect sign of cerebral venous thrombosis, i.e., the inverted flow direction in a patent vein acting as alternative drainage route, in this example the *right* SPS, insonated in its medial end, which seems orthograde in the pre-terminal segment (**a**) and inverted in the previous segment (**b**)

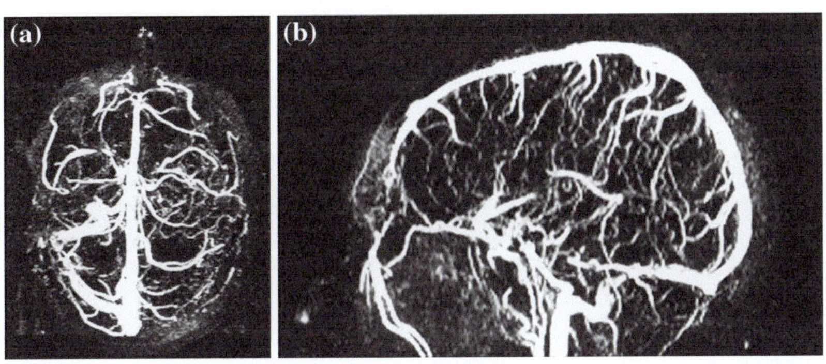

Fig. 7.5 Venous MRA with bidimensional reconstruction in a patient with cerebral venous thrombosis of the SRS, most of the GV and left TS

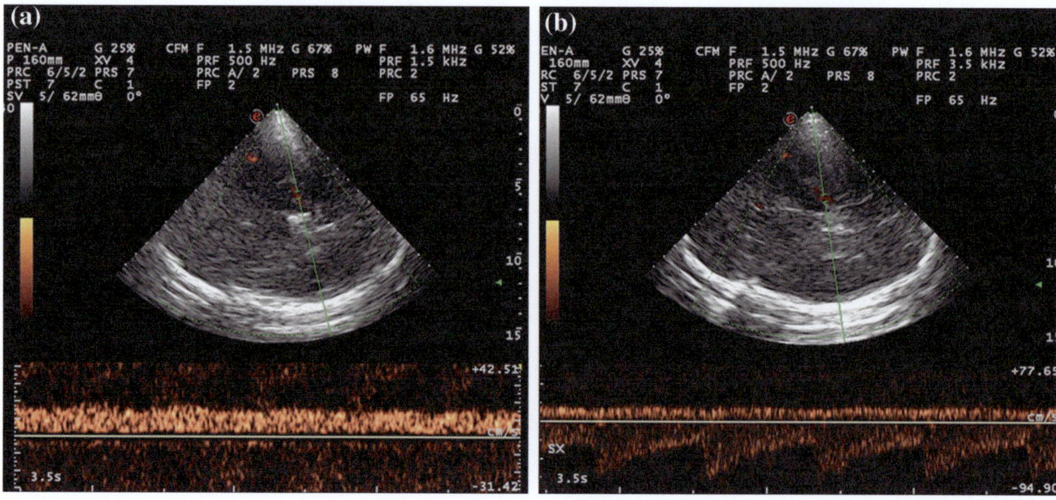

Fig. 7.6 **a** and **b** TCCS from the temporal bone window with insonation plane at the passage between mesencephalon and diencephalon in the same subject of the previous figure. It can be seen the post-peduncular segment of the BVR of both sides [the *right* BVR in the picture (**a**) and the *left* one in (**b**)] with inverted flow direction, congruent with the thrombotic occlusion of the GV-SRS

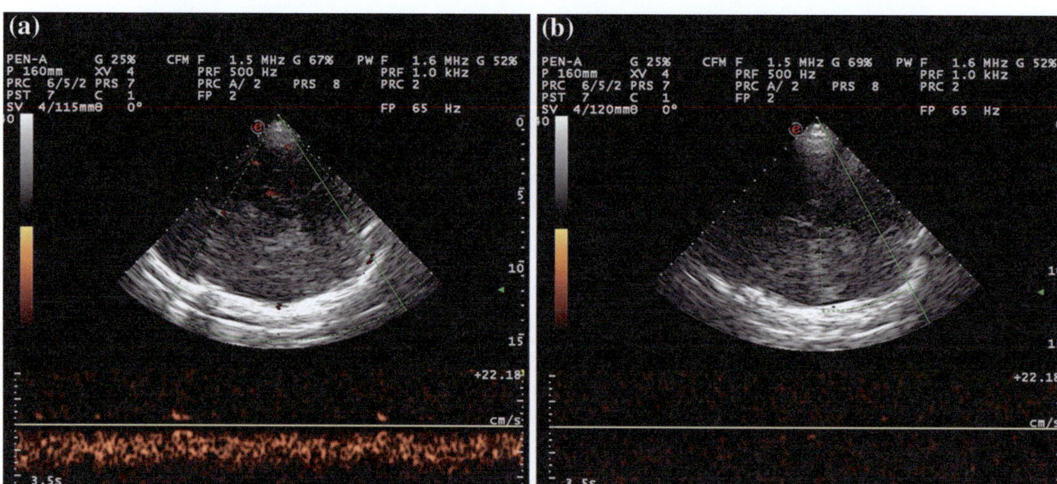

Fig. 7.7 **a** and **b** TCCS from temporal bone window in axial scan with midbrain insonation *plane*, oriented to the posterior cranial fossa (same subject of the previous two figures). Picture (**a**) shows the *right* TS, patent, and without abnormalities, (**b**) shows the site of *left* TS, lacking both for Doppler and for power-mode signals

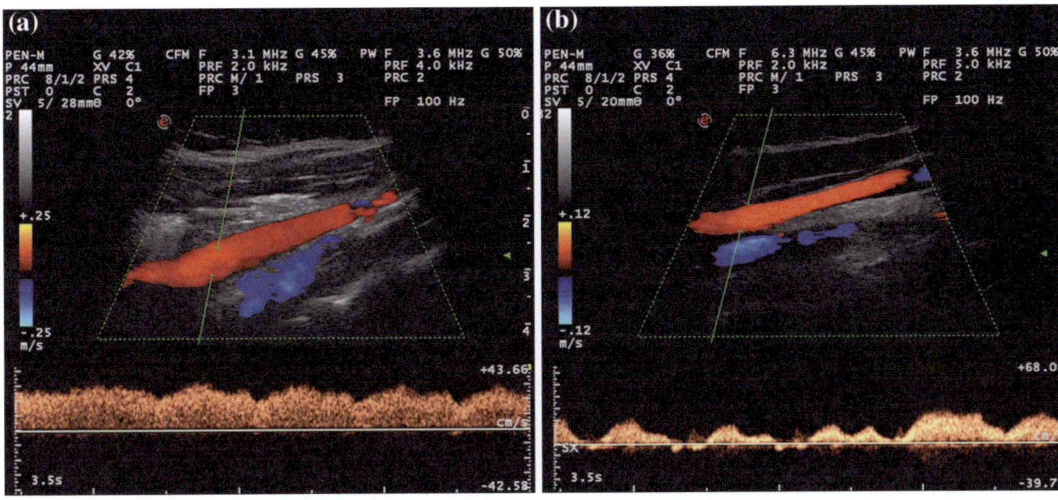

Fig. 7.8 Longitudinal scan of J3 IJV (same patients of the previous three figures). In picture (**a**), there is the *right* J3 IJV with a well-modulated Doppler waveform lacking abnormalities; in picture (**b**), there is the *left* J3 IJV, whose Doppler waveform is characterized by an alternating flow with superimposed phasic flow variations due to the breath cycle, both for the flow direction and for the velocity. As demonstrated in the picture, indirect signs can be seen at the level of the extracranial venous district, suggesting an intracranial site of disease, although these ones cannot be independently significant because of the wide variability of cerebral venous hemodynamics

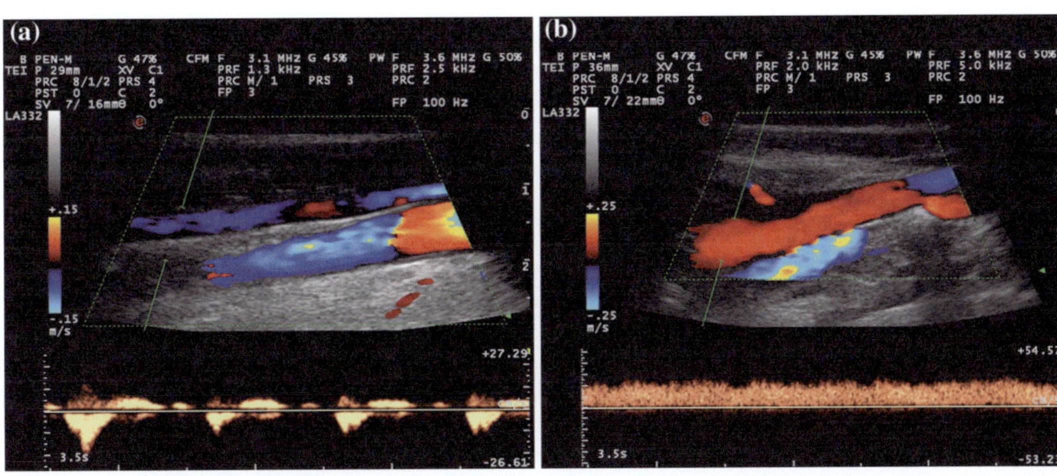

Fig. 7.9 Longitudinal scan of J2 IJV in Color mode in a patient with cerebral vein thrombosis involving the *left* TS. In picture (**a**), there is the *left* IJV with the corresponding Doppler waveform at alternating direction, phasic with the breath cycle (see also movies 7.6), while in picture (**b**), there is the *right* IJV, whose flow pattern is orthograde during the breath and heart cycles (see Movie 7.7)

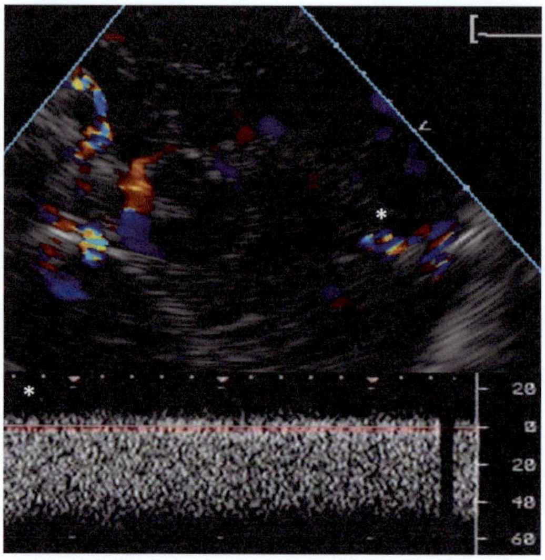

Fig. 7.10 TCCS from the right temporal bone window in axial scan, mesencephalic plane with posterior tilting of the probe, Color mode. The imaged patient has a severe TBI and a wide contusive injury with hemorrhagic evolution in the right brain hemisphere. It is possible to identify in Color mode the posterior end of the SRS with evident aliasing, as in the confluens of sinuses. The Doppler waveform corresponding to the SRS (*below*) shows an increased flow velocity and the loss of the regular pulsatility of the cerebral venous flow

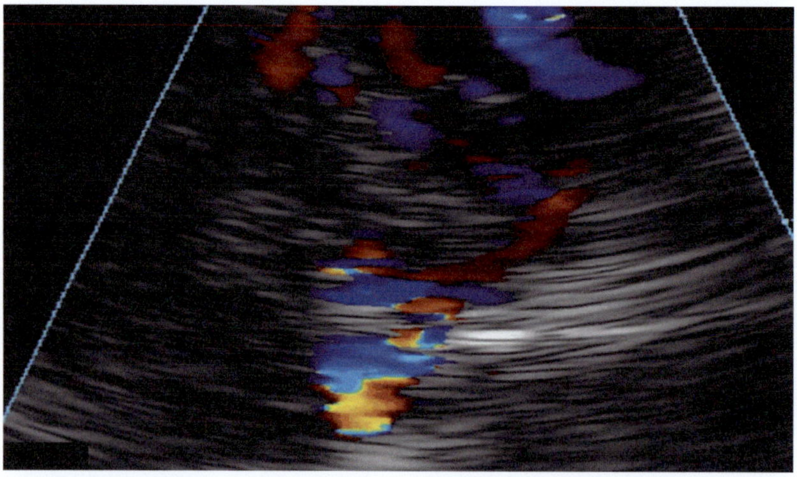

Fig. 7.11 TCCS from the right temporal bone window in axial scan, mesencephalic plane with posterior tilting of the probe, Color mode (same patient of the previous figure). Magnification of the confluens of sinuses and origin of the ipsilateral and contralateral TS. It is evident the aliasing effect on the contralateral TS compared with the ipsilateral one, as in the pre-terminal segment of the SRS

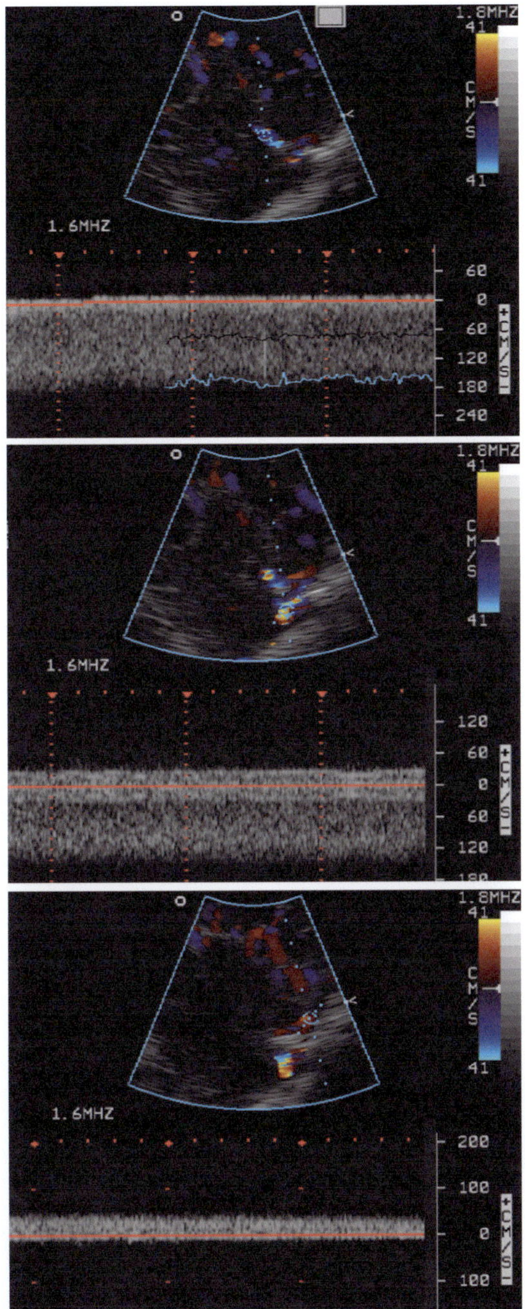

Fig. 7.12 TCCS from the *right* temporal bone window in axial scan, mesencephalic plane with posterior tilting of the probe, Color mode (same patient of the previous figures). Magnification of the confluens of sinuses and origin of the ipsilateral and contralateral TS. From *up to down*: Sampling of the Doppler waveform at the level of the pre-terminal segment of SRS with angle correction, showing the increased flow velocity corresponding to hyperflow condition. Sampling of the Doppler waveform at the level of the contralateral TS, showing similar flow features in comparison with the ipsilateral TS, associated with a marked turbulence signal. Sampling of the Doppler waveform at the level of the ipsilateral TS, showing a continuous, orthograde low flow velocity signal. It is likely that a flow diversion to the SRS-contralateral TS pathway is present, because of the intracranial hypertension with a mass effect from the cerebral right lesion, determining a decreased drainage on the ipsilateral TS

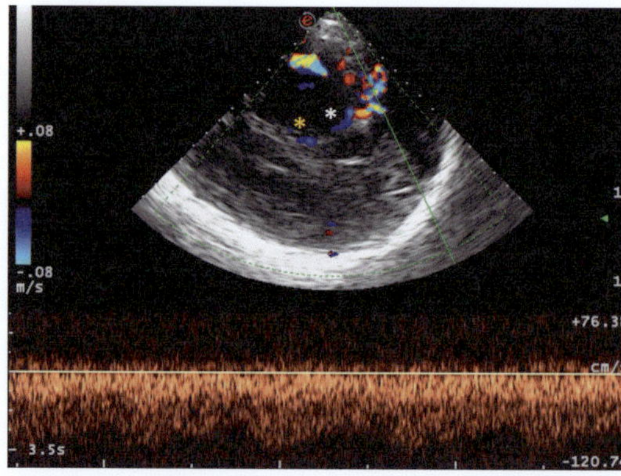

Fig. 7.13 TCCS from the temporal bone window on the diencephalic plane with posterior tilting of the probe. In Color mode, it is well evident the wide area of mosaic aliasing, corresponding to the nidus of an AVM with a parietal-occipital localization, fed by MCA branches and draining by an abnormal vein (*white asterisk*) to the GV (*yellow asterisk*). The flow waveform sampled on the nidus shows at least three different flow pathways, all with a "pseudoarterialized" morphology (see also Movies 7.8 and 7.9)

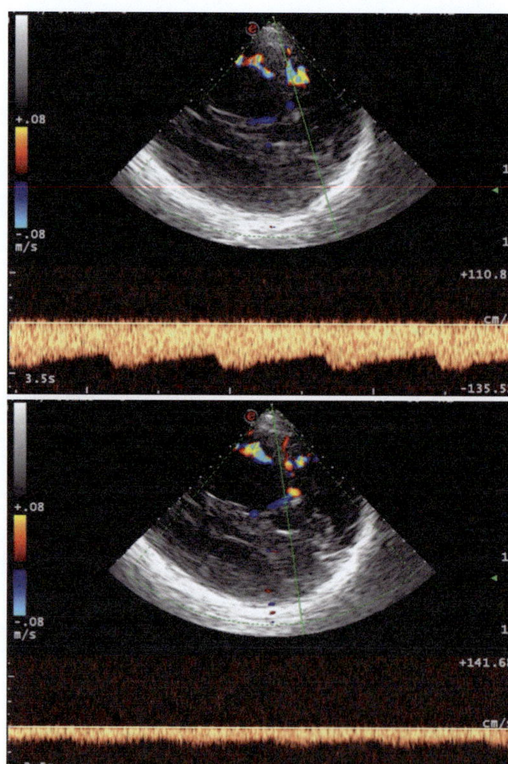

Fig. 7.14 TCCS, from the temporal bone window, on the diencephalic plane with posterior tilting of the probe (same patient of the previous figure). In the above image, the flow waveform features of one of the feeding arteries are shown; in the image below, the Doppler waveform of the main draining vein is shown with a pseudoarterializated morphology, before to go into the GV

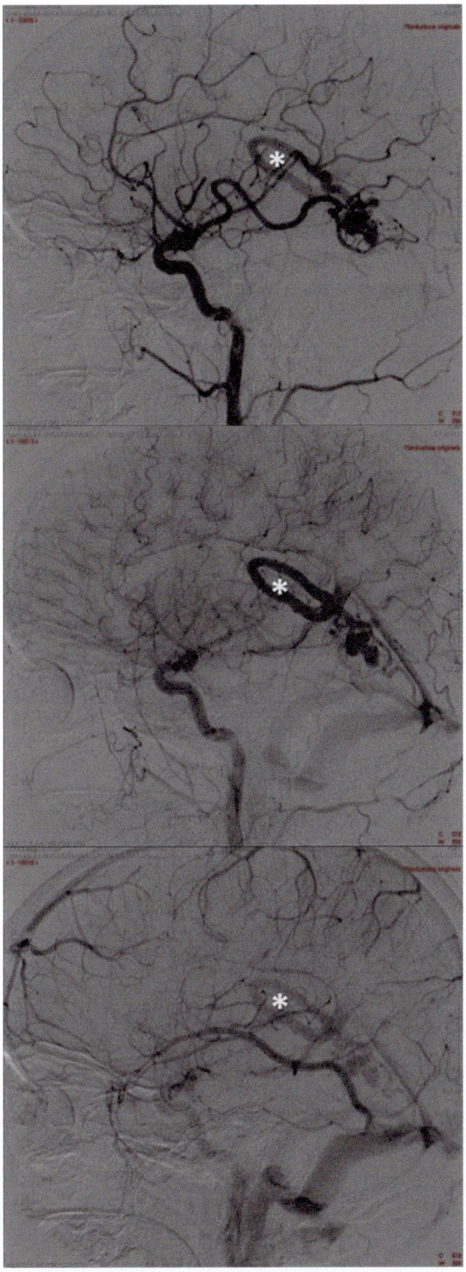

Fig. 7.15 Selective cerebral angiography (same patient of the previous two figures). It is evident an AVM located in the *right* anterior occipital region with a nidus of about 2.5 cm (maximum diameter). The main feeder comes from a branch of the right MCA, but minimal feeding comes also from PCA branches. The main drainage goes to the deep venous system through the GV, but a minor drainage pathway goes directly to the confluens of sinuses

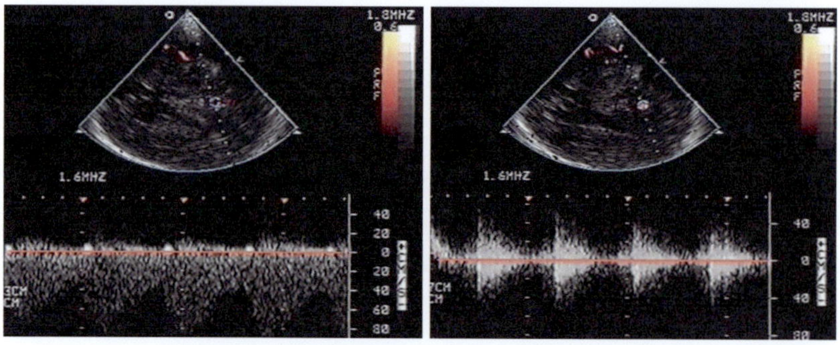

Fig. 7.16 TCCS from temporal bone window in axial access on the ventricular plane in patient with a FAV whose drainage involves the GV. It can be noted the increased flow velocity with high pulsatility pattern, arterial-like, on GV, imaged in an oblique ventricular plane (*upper* half of the figure; see also Movie 7.10), but slightly moving the sample volume it is found a markedly turbulent Doppler waveform, whose acoustic correlate is represented by "musical murmurs" (lower half of the picture; see also **Movie** 7.11)

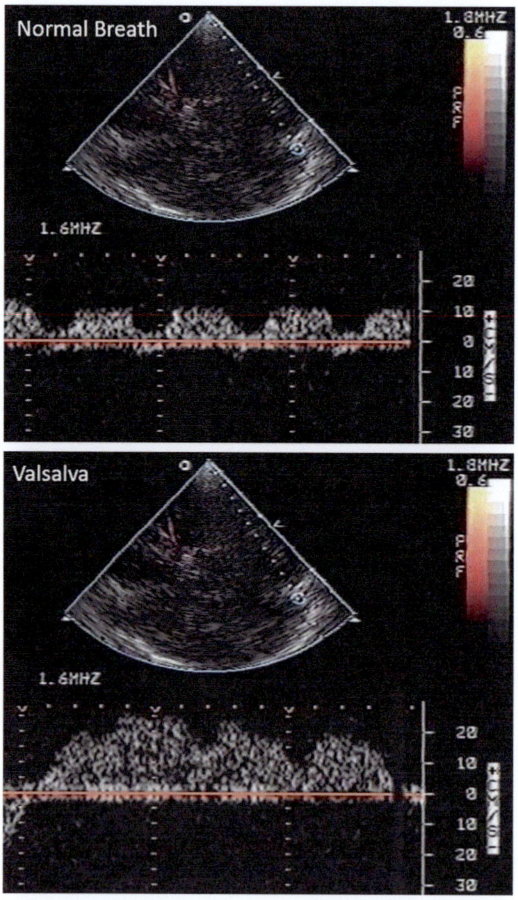

Fig. 7.17 TCCS from the temporal bone window, in axial scan, with an access for the posterior cranial fossa (same patient of the previous figure), showing the involvement of the TS of both sides as draining routes of the FAV. Indeed the *left* TS, imaged by a contralateral insonation, has a Doppler waveform with phasically inverted direction during normal breath and transient orthograde flow jet during the Valsalva maneuver, followed by a long-lasting phase of inverted flow direction

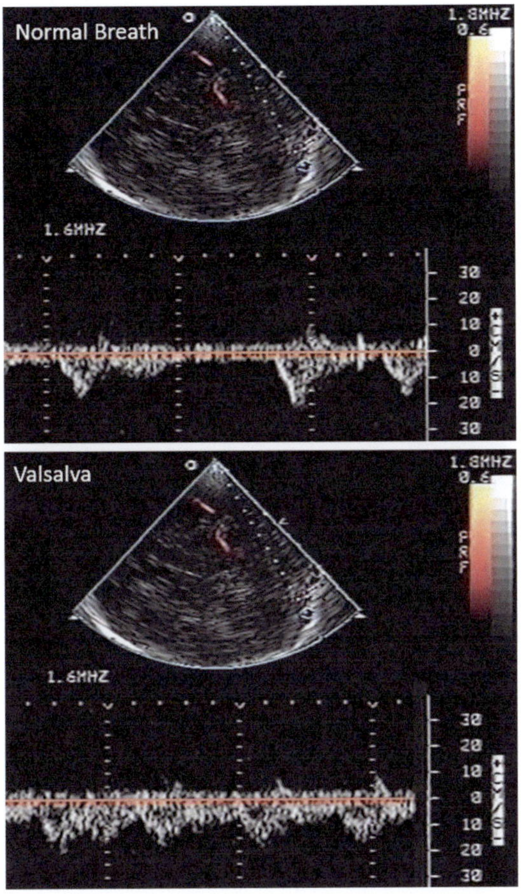

Fig. 7.18 TCCS from the temporal bone window, in axial scan, with an access for the posterior cranial fossa (same patient of the previous figure), showing the involvement of the TS of both sides as draining routes of the FAV. The *right* TS, imaged by a contralateral insonation approach, shows a Doppler waveform with an increased pulsatility index and orthograde direction during normal breath, but during the Valsalva maneuver, the pulsatility index decreases, maintaining the orthograde direction

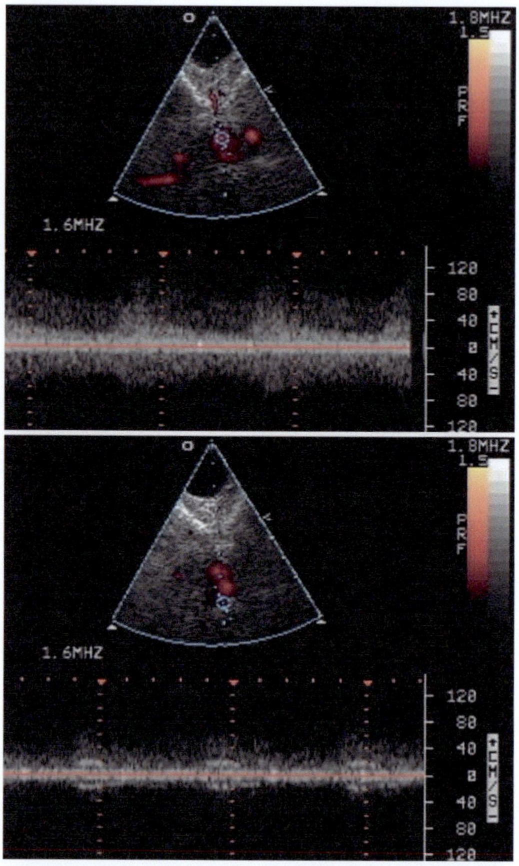

Fig. 7.19 TCCS from the ophthalmic window, Power mode in patient with a carotid-cavernous fistula. In the upper image is sampled the Doppler waveform at the nidus, in the retrobulbar region, along the ICA course; at least three flow routes are identified, and one of these has a venous aspect with a pseudoarterialized pattern (see also Movie 7.12). In the *lower* image, the arterio-venous communication is likely sampled, as signaled by the bidirectional harmonic artifact corresponding to the "musical murmurs" (see also Movie 7.13)

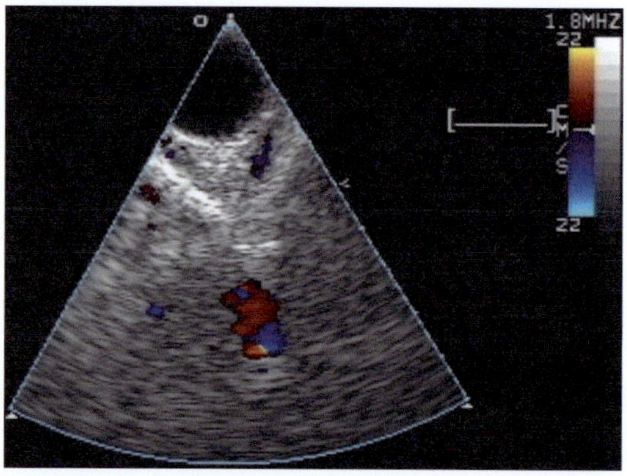

Fig. 7.20 TCCS from the ophthalmic window, Color mode in patient with a carotid-cavernous fistula (same patient of the previous figure). It is well evident the aliasing signal corresponding to the region depicted in power mode in the previous figure

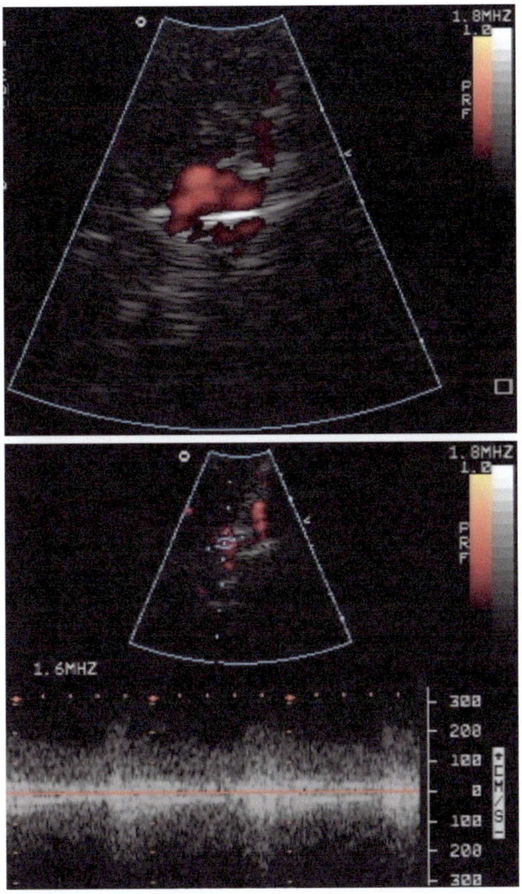

Fig. 7.21 TCCS from the temporal bone window, in coronal access on the carotid syphon in patient with a carotid cavernous fistula. In the upper image, there is a magnification of the carotid channel with a leakage of the Power signal outside its edges, in spite of the adequacy of the gain and the other setting items. In the *lower* image, there is the Doppler waveform, corresponding to the ICA with a bidirectional and turbulent flow (see also Movie 7.14)

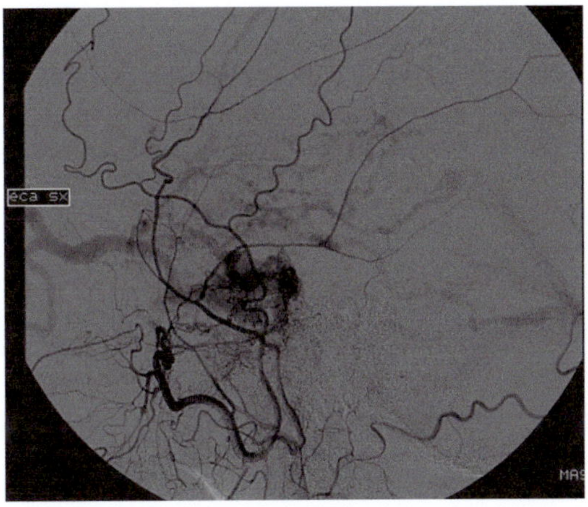

Fig. 7.22 Digital angiography of the same subject of the previous figure. It is well evident in the retroorbital region a network of several communicating vessels draining into the cavernous sinus

References

1. Valdueza JM, Schultz M, Harms L, Einhäupl KM (1995) Venous transcranial Doppler ultrasound monitoring in acute dural sinus thrombosis. Report of two cases. Stroke 26:1196–1199
2. Schreiber SJ, Stolz E, Valdueza JM (2002) Transcranial ultrasonography of cerebral veins and sinuses. Eur J Ultrasound 16:59–72
3. Stolz E, Gerriets T, Bodeker RH, Hugens-Penzel M, Kaps M (2002) Intracranial venous hemodynamics is a factor related to a favorable outcome in cerebral venous thrombosis. Stroke 33:1645–1650
4. Stolz E, Gerriets T, Babacan SS, Jauss M, Kraus J, Kaps M (2002) Intracranial venous hemodynamics in patients with midline dislocation due to postischemic brain edema. Stroke 33:479–485
5. Martin PJ, Gaunt ME, Naylor AR, Hope DT, Orpe V, Evans DH (1994) Intracranial aneurysms and arteriovenous malformations: transcranial colour-coded sonography as a diagnostic aid. Ultrasound Med Biol 20:689–698
6. Klötzsch C, Henkes H, Nahser HC, Kühne D, Berlit P (1995) Transcranial color-coded duplex sonography in cerebral arteriovenous malformations. Stroke 26:2298–2301
7. Baumgartner RW, Mattle HP, Schroth G (1996) Transcranial colour-coded duplex sonography of cerebral arteriovenous malformations. Neuroradiology 38:734–737
8. el-Saden SM, Grant EG, Sayre J, Vinuela F, Duckwiler G (1997) Transcranial color Doppler imaging of brain arteriovenous malformations in adults. J Ultrasound Med 16:327–334
9. Kaspera W, Majchrzak H (2002) Evaluation of blood supply dynamics and possibilities of cerebral arteriovenous malformations (AVM) imaging by means of transcranial color-coded duplex sonography (TCCS). Neurol Neurochir Pol 36:735–748
10. Arning C, Grzyska U, Lachenmayer L (1997) Lateral cranial dural fistula. Detection with Doppler and duplex ultrasound. Nervenarzt 68:139–146
11. Tsai LK, Jeng JS, Liu HM, Wang HJ, Yip PK (2004) Intracranial dural arteriovenous fistulas with or without cerebral sinus thrombosis: Analysis of 69 patients. J Neurol Neurosurg Psychiatry 75:1639–1641
12. Baumgartner RW, Gönner F, Arnold M, Müri RM (1997) Transtemporal power- and frequency-based color-coded duplex sonography of cerebral veins and sinuses. AJNR Am J Neuroradiol 18:1771–1781
13. Chen YW, Jeng JS, Liu HM, Yip PK, Hwang BS, Lin WH, Chang YC, Tu YK (1996) Diagnosis and followup of carotid-cavernous fistulas by carotid duplex sonography and transcranial color Doppler imaging. Ultrasound Med Biol 22:1155–1162
14. Schreiber SJ, Diehl RR, Weber W, Henkes H, Nahser HC, Lehmann R, Doepp F, Valdueza JM (2004) Doppler sonographic evaluation of shunts in patients with dural arteriovenous fistulas. AJNR Am J Neuroradiol 25:775–780
15. Harrer JU, Popescu O, Henkes HH, Klötzsch C (2005) Assessment of dural arteriovenous fistulae by transcranial color-coded duplex sonography. Stroke 36:976–979
16. Lin HJ, Yip PK, Liu HM, Hwang BS, Chen RC (1994) Noninvasive hemodynamic classification of carotid-cavernous sinus fistulas by duplex carotid sonography. J Ultrasound Med 13:105–113
17. Chen YW, Jeng JS, Liu HM, Hwang BS, Lin WH, Yip PK (2000) Carotid and transcranial color-coded duplex sonography in different types of carotid-cavernous fistula. Stroke 31:701–706

8 Global Hemodynamic Evaluation and Outflow Variability

It is well known that the two main pathways of cerebral venous outflow are the jugular and the vertebral axis, with a predominance of the former in supine position and an activation of the latter during upright position and in the sitting position [1].

Such conformation, demonstrated by physiological studies and mathematical models and considered as paradigmatic of the normal behavior of cerebral venous drainage, is not, however, the only possibility that can be identified in healthy subjects. As a side effect of the large variety of the anatomic conformation of the main outflow veins and of the anastomotic connections, there is furthermore the possibility of several functional variations of the cerebral venous outflow up to the almost complete dependence on extrajugular and extravertebral veins. Nevertheless, this does not necessarily imply ascertained and demonstrated pathological consequences.

More specifically, the mathematical model devised by Gisolf et al. [1] on the basis of experiments performed with ultrasound methodologies on healthy voluntaries, took into account the existence of a single alternative outflow besides the jugular axis, i.e., the vertebral venous system. As a result, the part of the blood volume that was not accounted for at the jugular level in the standing and sitting position was automatically allocated to the vertebral system. Gisolf's model has nonetheless mathematically confirmed the dependence on posture of the cerebral venous outflow, as already detected in healthy subjects [2]. It has, however, been well known for a long time in the literature that the bilateral dissection of the internal jugular vein at cervical level does not determine the impairment of the cerebral venous outflow [3]. The studies of Valdueza et al. [4] both on ultrasound imaging and on neuroradiological imaging have shown a greater variety of behavior of the cerebral venous outflow in healthy subjects with different drainage patterns.

In the above-mentioned study, three different drainage patterns have been put forward on the basis of the behavior identified in 15 healthy subjects:

- Type I: blood volume carried by the jugular veins for more than 2/3 of the whole arterial inflow;
- Type II: blood volume carried by the jugular veins amounting to between 1/3 and 2/3 of the whole arterial inflow;
- Type III: blood volume carried by the jugular veins amounting to less than 1/3 of the whole arterial inflow.

Type I is the so-called jugular drainer, whereas types II and III are the "extra-jugular drainers," which, on the basis of the simultaneous RMN findings, may be further divided into a subgroup of "neck drainers" by means of the deep cervical veins and of "spinal drainers" through the cervical epidural venous plexus.

From the anatomic point of view, the role and the varying activation of these extrajugular and extravertebral veins had been previously pointed out in normal and pathological situations. In

G. Malferrari et al., *Neurosonological Evaluation of Cerebral Venous Outflow*,
DOI: 10.1007/978-88-470-5465-3_8, © Springer-Verlag Italia 2014

particular, the intra- and extraspinal venous system does not involve only the cervical area but it stretches out along the whole length of the spine in a network of vessels without valves in which the direction of the flux may show dynamic changes according to the pressure gradient [5].

As stated by Valdueza et al. [4], Batson had already pointed out in the 1940s [6] that the total amount of the cross-sectional area of the non-jugular veins at the level of the cranial base exceeds the jugular veins one. The total volume capacity of the non-jugular ways has been calculated to be equal to 1,000 ml [7], which is anyhow sufficient to guarantee the whole cerebral venous drainage by itself.

At the level of the cranial base and of the atlanto-occipital joint, the condylar venous system represents an efficient anastomotic channel that lets the flow volume move from the jugular venous system to the intraspinal vertebral one, as well as to the deep cervical vein system. The latter may, however, receive part of the jugular drainage also through the occipital veins which outflow from the sinuses confluence by means and through the mastoid vein outflowing from the TS-SyS.

In such a general context, characterized by anatomic and functional variability, the border between normality and pathologic venous outflow appears to be difficult to identify. In the following images, the ultrasound study of cerebral venous outflow and its pitfalls will be illustrated (Table 8.1).

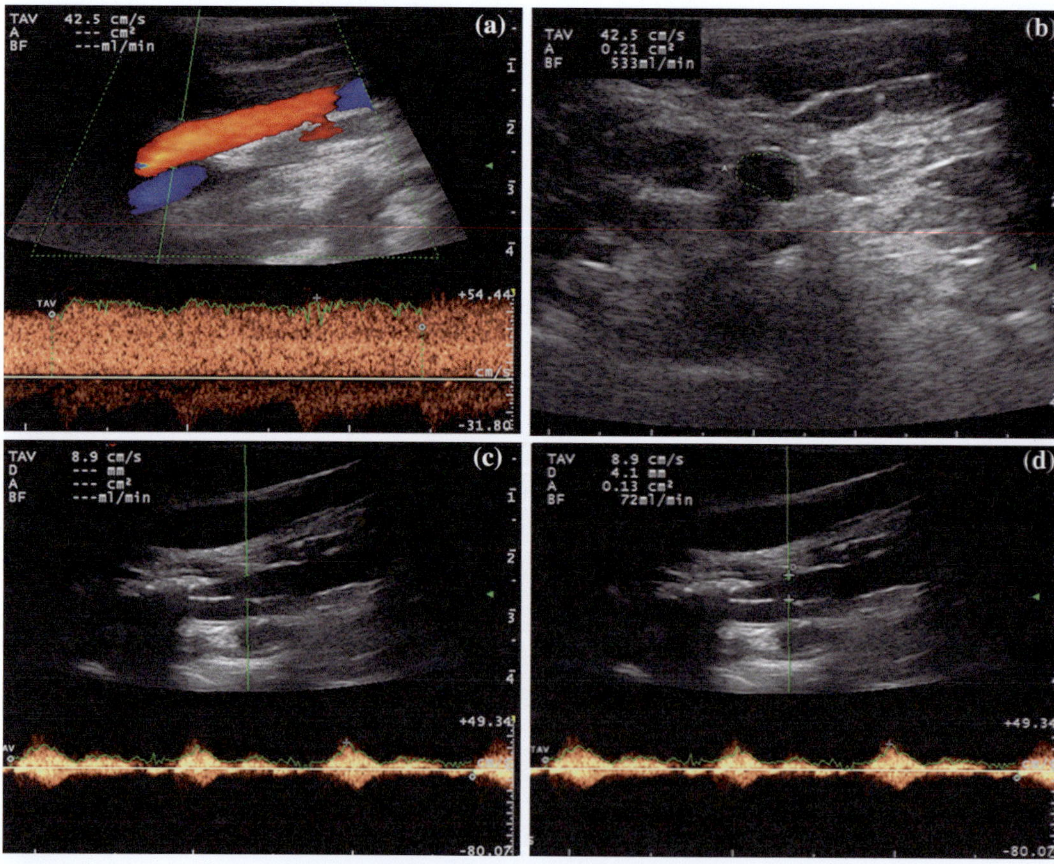

Fig. 8.1 Example of cerebral venous outflow measurement in supine position on the *right side*. **a** J3 IJV Doppler sampling and TAV measurement. **b** J3 JJV CSA measurement and automatic blood flow calculation in ml/min. **c** V1 VV Doppler sampling and TAV measurement. **d** V1 VV diameter measurement and automatic CSA and blood flow calculation

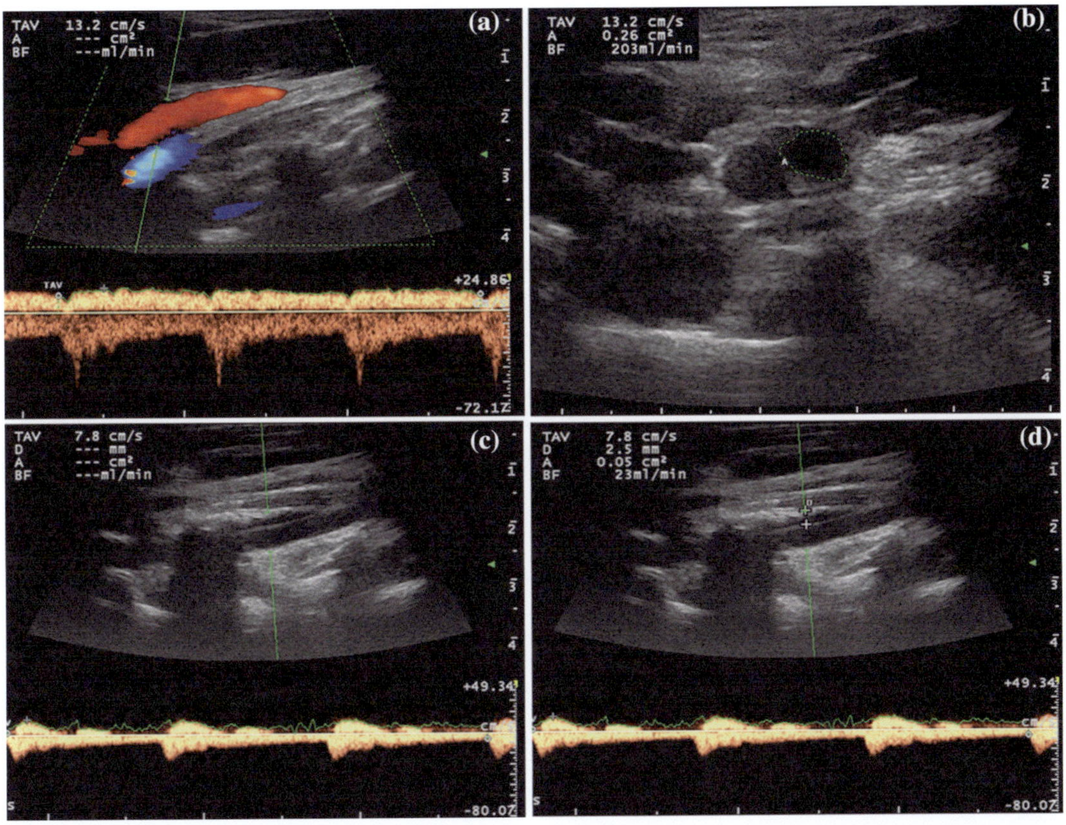

Fig. 8.2 Example of cerebral venous outflow measurement in supine position on the *left side*. **a** J3 IJV Doppler sampling and TAV measurement. **b** J3 IJV CSA measurement and automatic blood flow calculation in ml/min. **c** V1 VV Doppler sampling and TAV measurement. **d** V1 VV diameter measurement and automatic CSA and blood flow calculation

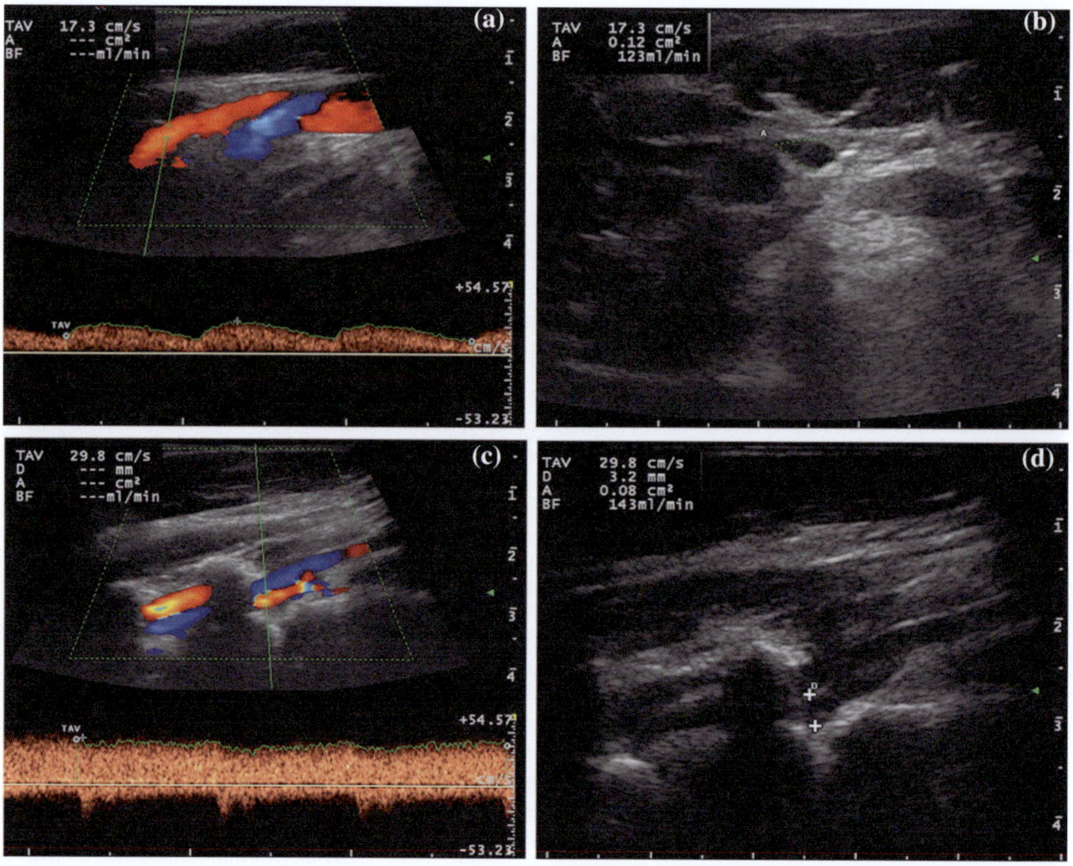

Fig. 8.3 Example of cerebral venous outflow measurement in upright position on the *right side*. **a** J3 IJV Doppler sampling and TAV measurement. **b** J3 IJV CSA measurement and automatic blood flow calculation in ml/min. **c** V1 VV Doppler sampling and TAV measurement. **d** V1 VV diameter measurement and automatic CSA and blood flow calculation

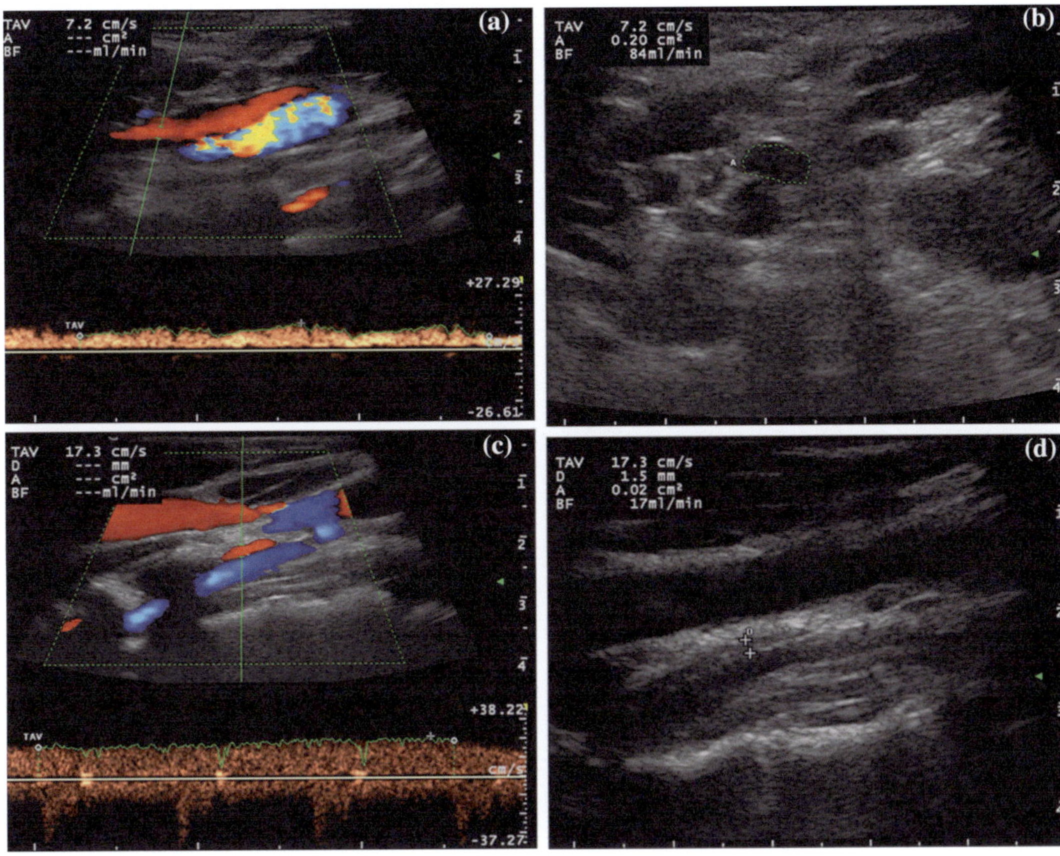

Fig. 8.4 Example of cerebral venous outflow measurement in *upright* position on the *left side*. **a** J3 IJV Doppler sampling and TAV measurement. **b** J3 IJV CSA measurement and automatic blood flow calculation in ml/min. **c** V1 VV Doppler sampling and TAV measurement. **d** V1 VV diameter measurement and automatic CSA and blood flow calculation

Table 8.1 Summary of the outflow measurements

	Blood flow in supine position (ml/min)	Blood flow in upright position (ml/min)
Right J3 IJV	533	123
Right V1 VV	72	143
Left J3 IJV	203	84
Left V1 VV	23	17

References

1. Gisolf J, van Lieshout JJ, van Heusden K, Pott F, Stok WJ, Karemaker JM (2004) Human cerebral venous outflow pathway depends on posture and central venous pressure. J Physiol 560:317–327
2. Valdueza JM, von Munster T, Hoffman O et al (2000) Postural dependency of the cerebral venous outflow. Lancet 355:200–201
3. Gius JA, Grier DH (1950) Venous adaptation following bilateral radical neck dissection with excision of the jugular vein. Surgery 28:305–321
4. Doepp F, Schreiber SJ, von Munster T et al (2004) How does the blood leave the brain? A systematic ultrasound analysis of cerebral venous drainage patterns. Neuroradiology 46:565–570
5. Chou CH, Chao AC, Hu HH (2002) Ultrasonographic evaluation of vertebral venous valves. AJNR Am J Neuroradiol 23(8):1418–1420
6. Batson OV (1944) Anatomical problems concerned in the study of cerebral blood flow. Fed Proc 3:139–144
7. Eckenhoff JE (1970) The physiologic significance of the vertebral venous plexus. Surg Gynecol Obst 131:72–78

9 Imaging Fusion Technology for Evaluating Intracranial Veins

The technology of the real-time imaging fusion has been devised and applied to different body regions and pathological situations; it has been developed through the combination of multiple imaging modalities, and in its extreme evolution, it has become a veritable virtual navigator. Its aim is to combine a static modality and a dynamic modality. The static, but with high spatial resolution mode, modality has been previously acquired and incorporated on the platform of the browser; the dynamic mode is executed directly on the patient using the anatomical guidance of the first modality formerly uploaded. The second imaging modality has dynamic characteristics that make it a high temporal resolution tool, but with less pronounced spatial resolution. The purpose of the imaging fusion is to combine the high spatial with the high temporal resolution, which are not available together in the same method. In this way, the information of the two methods is blended so as to obtain a real-time reconstruction of the examined structures. In fact, the rationale of this technology is to realize a real virtual navigation, in order to allow better identification of the parenchymal and vascular structures; furthermore, this technology is useful in some therapeutic applications, such as the percutaneous treatment for focal lesions in the liver.

Typically, the first imaging modality, which has been previously acquired on the patient, sometimes with the skin application of precise landmarks, is usually the computerized axial tomography or magnetic resonance imaging, whereas the second imaging mode, in real time, is an ultrasound technique.

This strategy allows not only a precise real-time anatomical mapping of the parenchyma and the structures explored by ultrasound, but also the direct volumetric investigation of the structures. This is performed by scanning, often with oblique, unconventional planes, the three-dimensional imaging reconstruction of the organ when examined by means of the first imaging modality.

Initially, the applications of this investigation modality have been extracerebral, beginning, as it could be expected, with organs easy to be studied by ultrasound because of the absence of bone wall. The first organs studied were the abdominal parenchyma (for example, liver, spleen) and subsequently organs as the prostate, the breast, and the thyroid [1]. The goal of applying the virtual navigation technology to these organs was the therapeutic outcome, for

Electronic supplementary material Supplementary material is available in the online version of this chapter at http://dx.doi.org/10.1007/978-88-470-5465-3_9. Videos can also be accessed at http://www.springerimages.com/videos/978-88-470-5465-3

G. Malferrari et al., *Neurosonological Evaluation of Cerebral Venous Outflow*,
DOI: 10.1007/978-88-470-5465-3_9, © Springer-Verlag Italia 2014

example the percutaneous treatment for focal hepatic lesions under ultrasound guidance, often with the help of ultrasound contrast [2, 3]. The application of this method to the study of cerebral parenchymal structures and intracranial circulation is much more recent. In this area, the last frontier was the study of the intracranial venous district, which has allowed to propose and validate innovative study approaches, such as the evaluation of the transverse sinus (TS) ipsilateral to the temporal window insonation [4, 5].

The imaging fusion of the two modes is possible thanks to an electromagnetic tracking system, which defines the correspondence between the images from the first imaging modality preloaded on an ultrasound platform and those of the second imaging modality. The second images are acquired in real time, either through the skin landmarks corresponding to the ones used in the planning phase of the study with the first mode, or through the manual identification of the planes of image correspondence between the two modes. In order to make this possible, the ultrasound probe is integrated with an electromagnetic tracking system within a magnetic field of very low power and flow, generated by a magnet connected with the system.

The stages of the study with the virtual navigation are substantially as follows:

- Implementation of the study with the first imaging modality (CT or MRI), with or without skin landmarks
- Loading of such DICOM format images on the ultrasound platform and selection of the appropriate sequence in order to enable the software to perform the volumetric reconstruction
- Carrying out of the ultrasound study through a selection of the scanning planes corresponding to the virtual scans in the recreated volume. This step can be partly automated by means of the repositioning of cutaneous landmarks. The tracking system is set so as to recognize their spatial coordinates, within which ultrasound probe is made to move in an integral way with the electromagnetic tracking system. Another possibility is to proceed manually through the identification of the planes in the two imaging modalities. The precise control of the bony, parenchymal, and vascular landmarks ensures a perfect match between the planes and any subsequent adjustments
- Checking of the correspondence by means of the imaging of the arterial structures of the polygon of Willis
- Performing of the ultrasound study with the help of volumetric CT/MRI anatomical information on the screen and in virtual slicing on the basis of the ultrasound transducer movement.

In our experience on the manual identification of planes, if on the one hand it requires greater knowledge of the intracranial ultrasound anatomy, it is more flexible and easily manageable in the adjustment and correction phase during the examination on the other hand. It also allows the use of previous neuroimaging studies on the subject, which have not been specifically acquired in a dedicated manner and with the purpose of acting as first imaging modality for the virtual navigator. This can also be useful for short-term planning studies or in urgency.

The use of this technology permits to increase the rate of insonation of some venous structures that with previous approaches demonstrated to have a greater variability, such as the TS (this objective can be reached through the combination of the ipsilateral and contralateral insonation) [4, 5]. In fact, even in conditions of suboptimal insonation, it is possible to exploit the anatomical landmarks obtained with the first imaging modality for the search of the vessel under study. This is carried out through the sampling of the Doppler waveform, without taking up any analysis channels employed for the color mode or the power mode, which are not always effective as a guide for sampling the Doppler waveform.

The following figures show some examples of the practical application of this technique.

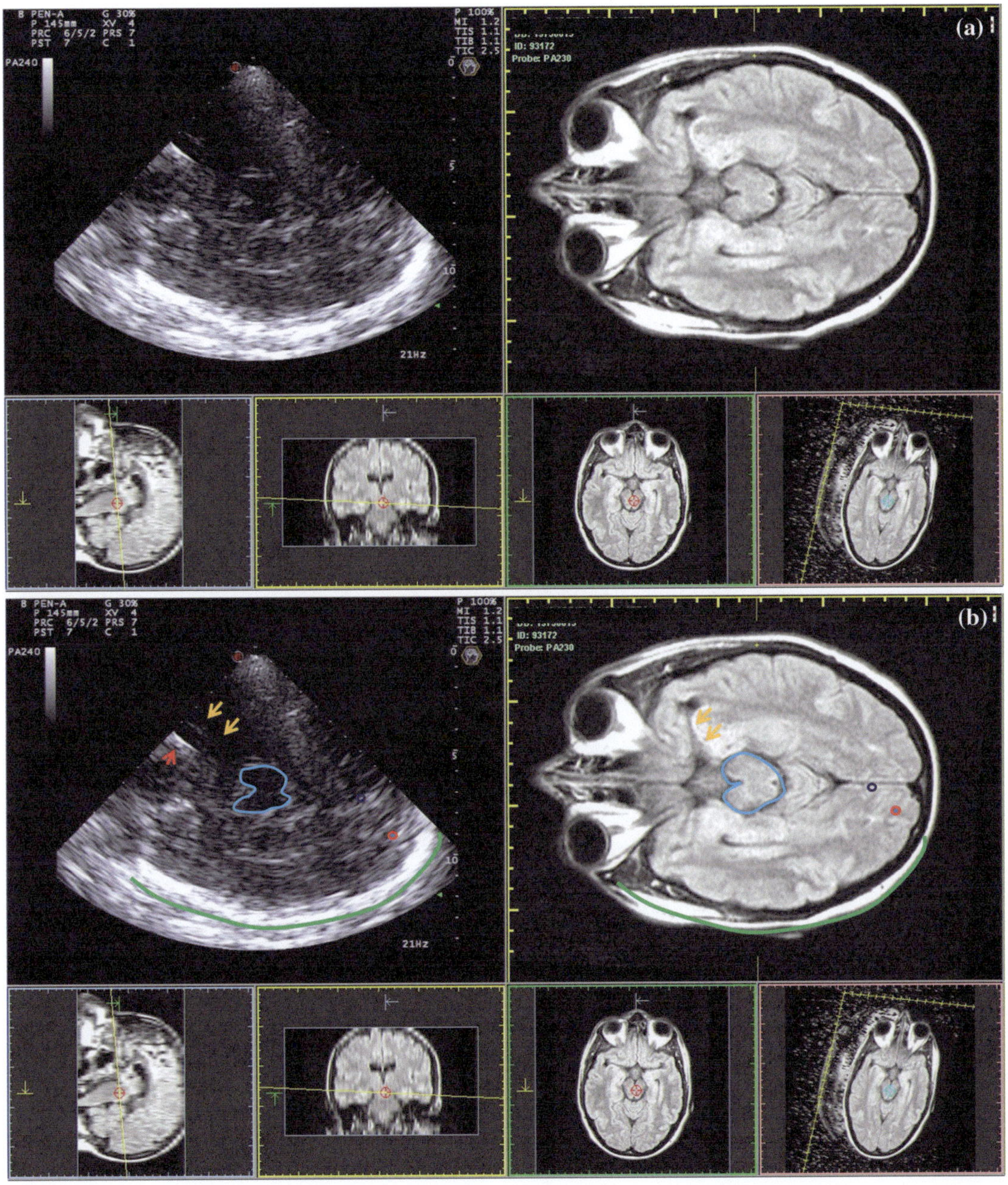

Fig. 9.1 In (**a**) it is possible to see an application of the virtual navigator method with the achievement of a full correspondence between anatomical TCCS and MRI as regards the parenchymal and bony landmarks of the mesencephalic plan. (**b**) Highlights the anatomical landmarks known to facilitate the interpretation and identification of the correspondences. On the top left of the screenshot TCCS is shown in the axial scan from the temporal window on the mesencephalic plan. At the front, the olfactory conduits are emphasized; they are located in the paramedian position below the hyperechogenicity of the small wing of the sphenoid bone (*red arrow*). This bony landmark is the identification reference of the middle cerebral artery, whose parietal interface is easily identifiable (*yellow arrows*, with the corresponding location on MRI). The contralateral skull is outlined in *green*, both on the TCCS and on MRI. The contour of the mesencephalon in section is instead outlined in *blue* on the two images. A *red ring* indicates the occipital pole contralateral to the site of insonation, while a *blue ring* marks the hyperechogenicity of the falx cerebri and the corresponding location of the falx on the axial MRI image. In the *lower part* of the screenshot, the reconstructed volume of RMN stands out, with the virtual scan plane corresponding to the ultrasonic one

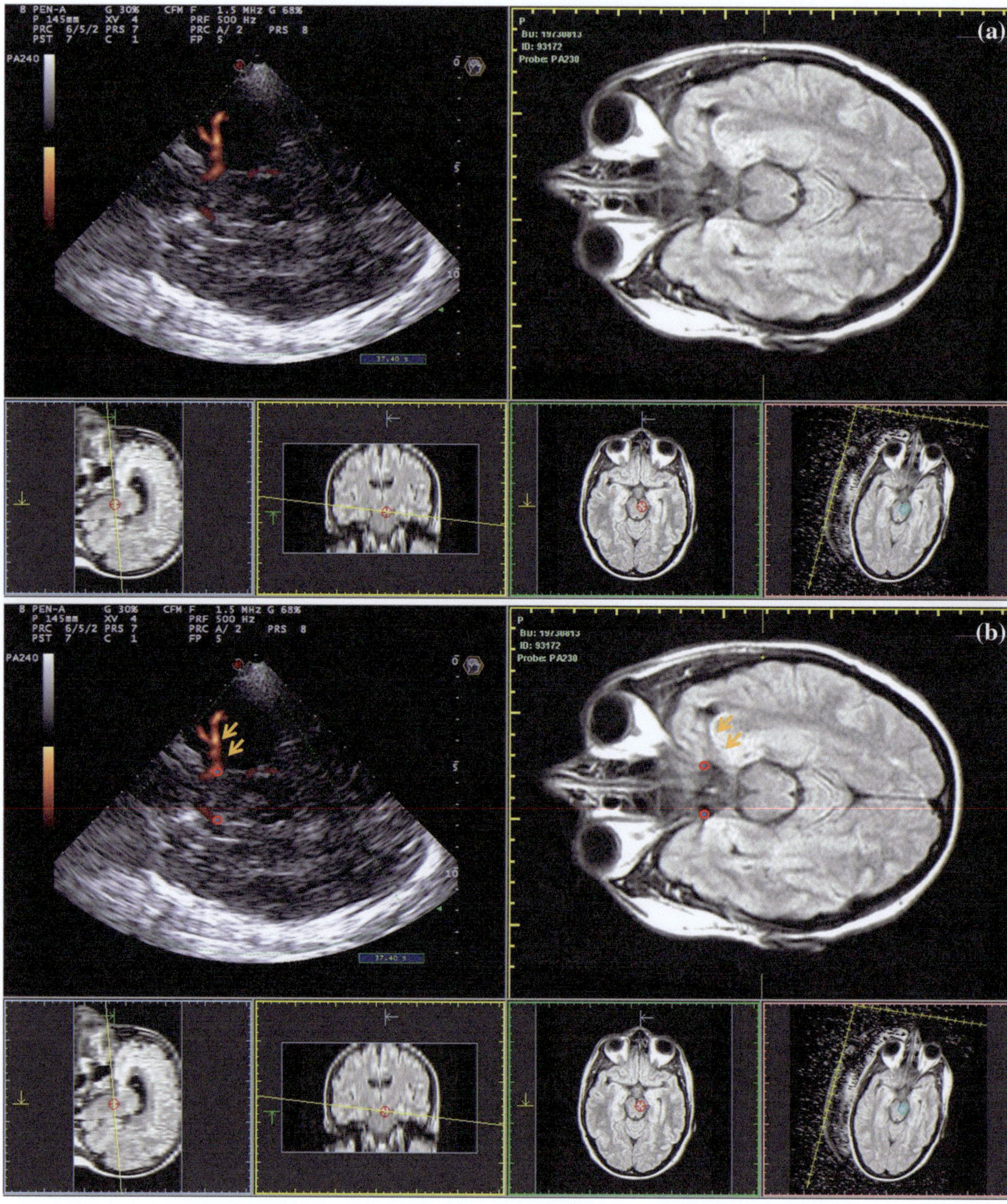

Fig. 9.2 **a**, **b** In the same way as in Fig. 9.1, this image confirms the correct identification of the middle cerebral artery course through the hyperechoic interface as the parallel track of its wall in the subarachnoid space (*yellow arrows* in **b**). The outflow of the internal carotid artery that forks into the MCA and the ACA (*red ring*) is also highlighted

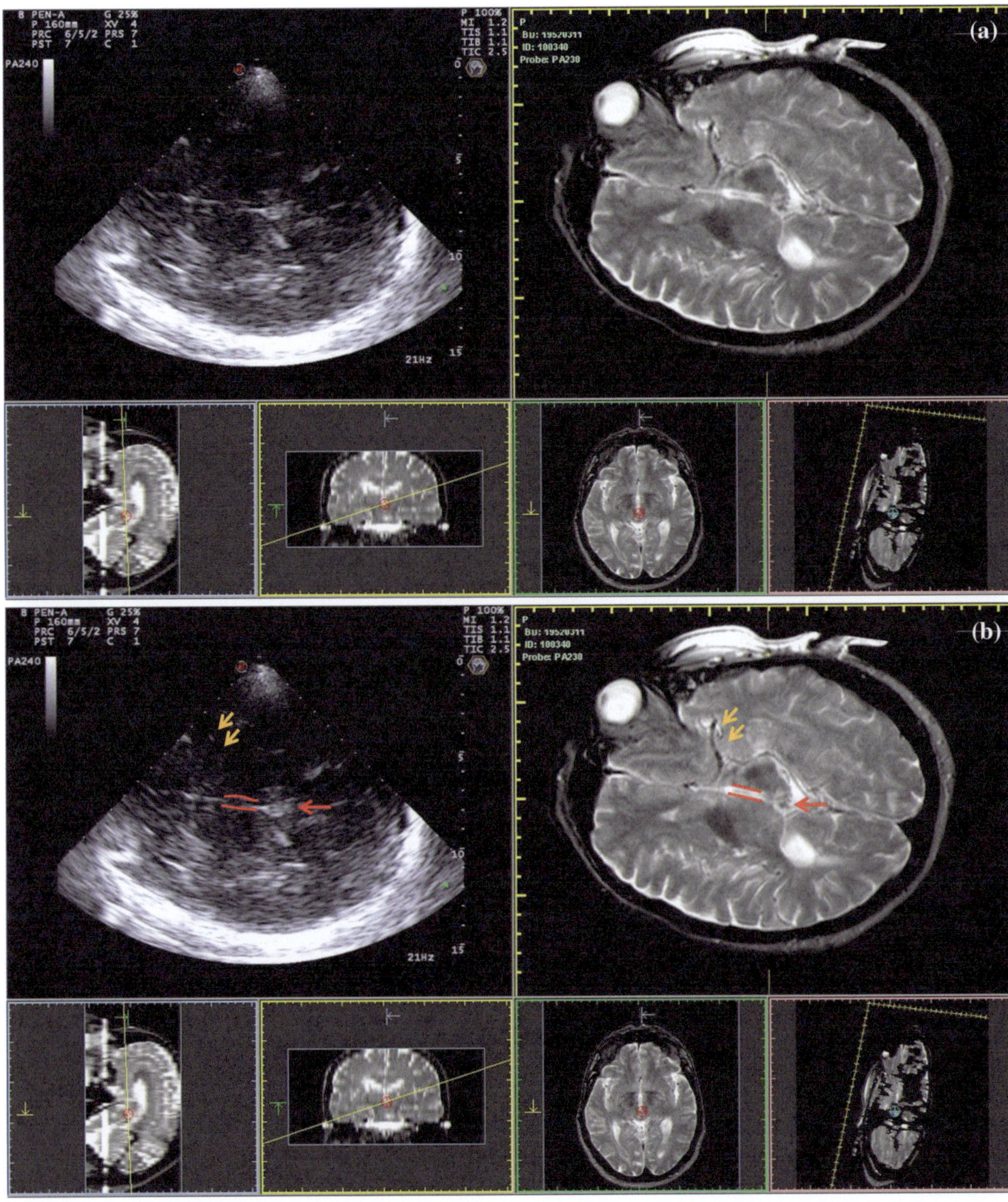

Fig. 9.3 In (**a**), it is possible to see an application of the virtual navigator method with the achievement of a full correspondence between anatomical TCCS and NMR as regards the parenchymal and bony landmarks of the diencephalic plan. In (**b**), the anatomical landmarks known to facilitate interpretation and identification of correspondences are highlighted. At the *top* of the screen to the *left*, TCCS in the axial scan from the temporal window on the diencephalic plan is shown. The parallel track image of the third ventricle, limited at the back from the hyperechogenicity of the epiphysis, is evident in the midline. The thalamus and caudate–lenticular complex are located close to the third ventricle. It is possible to see the parietal interface of the distal M1 segment and of M1-M2 transition of the MCA. (**b**) The same structures are evident, but they are outlined for an easy identification both in the ultrasound scan and in the oblique MRI brain image. The third ventricle is outlined in *red*, the epiphysis is indicated by a *red arrow*, and the interface of the MCA walls is marked with *yellow arrows*

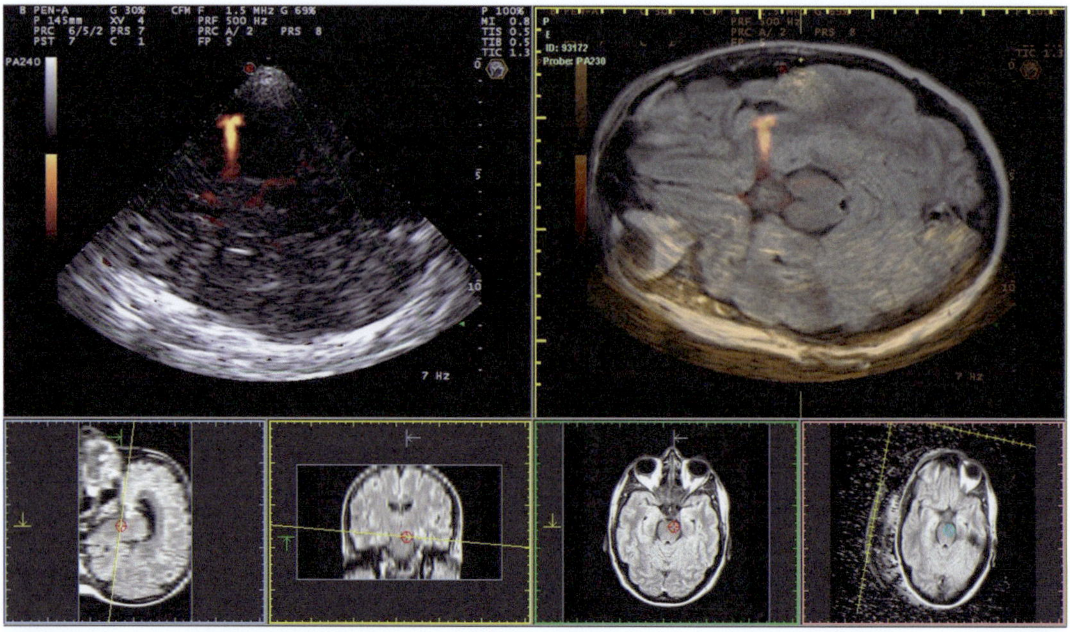

Fig. 9.4 On the screen, the precise overlap between the ultrasound and the corresponding MRI image of the mesencephalic plane is highlighted; MCA is displayed in power mode. In particular, note the course of the MCA that goes to the subarachnoid space, the contralateral skull which perfectly surrounds the contralateral temporal lobe, and the mesencephalic echoic profile that perfectly fits the MRI one

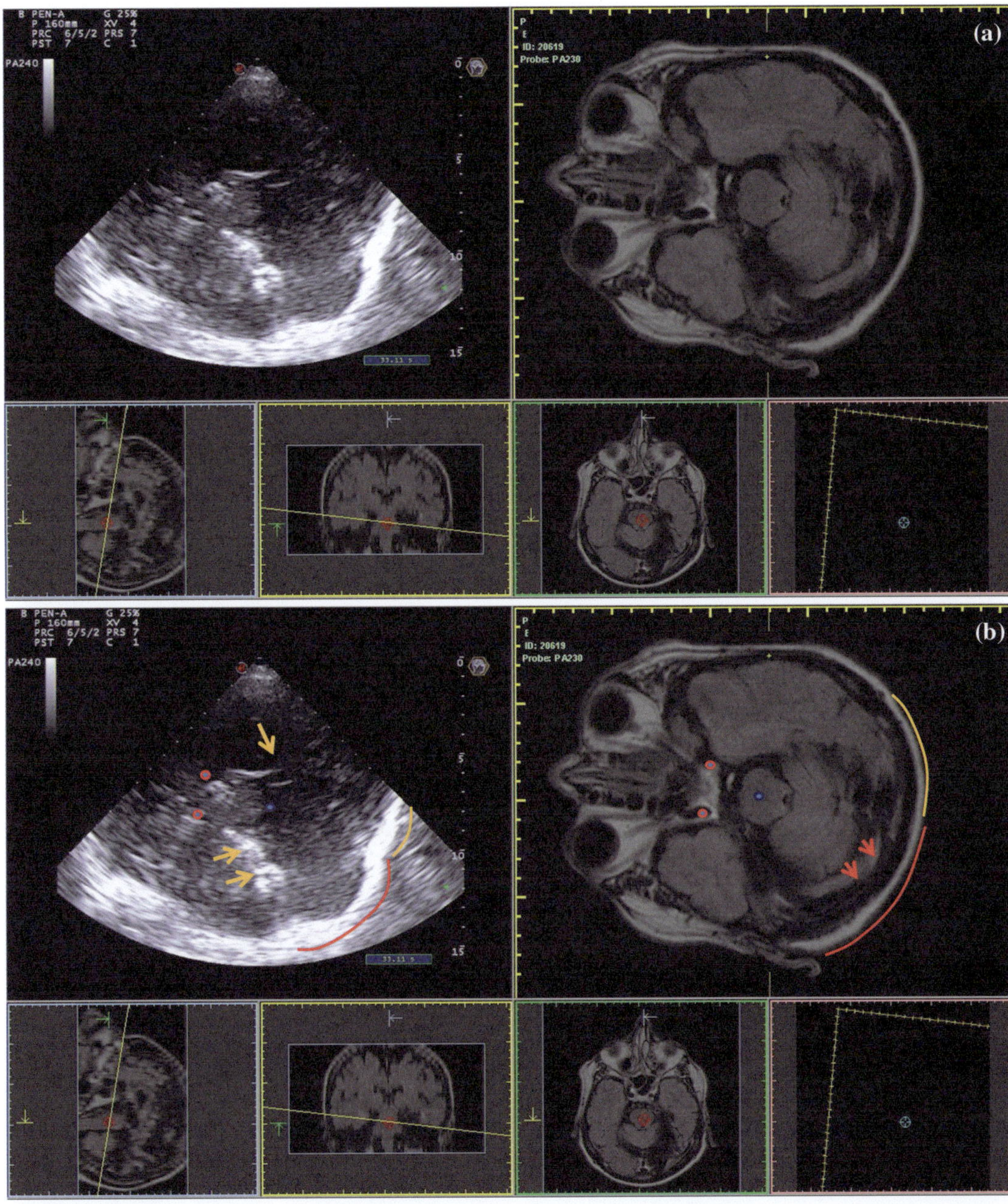

Fig. 9.5 (**a**) shows a further approach, with the comparison with the corresponding oblique MRI plane. It is useful for the parenchymal study but in particular for the study of the ipsilateral TS, i.e., the approach with access to the posterior fossa. In fact, the ultrasound image appears more oblique, with the display of both the ipsilateral and contralateral occipital skull at the level of the conduit course of the TS. The bony border landmarks of the posterior cranial fossa stand out: They are the contralateral and ipsilateral (only the medial segment) edge of the petrosal bone. The parenchymal access is pontine, as may be seen by MRI, and the horizontal part of the ICA is well detectable. In (**b**), the most important identifiable structures are well detailed and labeled to make them easier to be recognized. The ipsilateral occipital skull is shown in *yellow*, the contralateral skull is shown in *red*, and the conduit course of the TS is indicated by *red arrows* in the MRI. The contralateral and ipsilateral edge of the petrosal bone is indicated by *yellow arrows*, while the pons is marked by a *blue ring* and the horizontal part of the ICA by a *red ring*. In this case, it is clearly evident how the application of the imaging fusion technology allows the exploration of unusual approaches for the study of the brain parenchyma and vessels. In this way, the possibility of insonation of some structures is generally improved and the anatomy ultrasound finds a perfect match in a virtual plan equivalent to neuroradiological imaging, which is usually not explored. This approach also allows the examiner to acquire more familiarity with the ultrasound anatomy and therefore to improve the accuracy of insonation also when not using the virtual navigation system

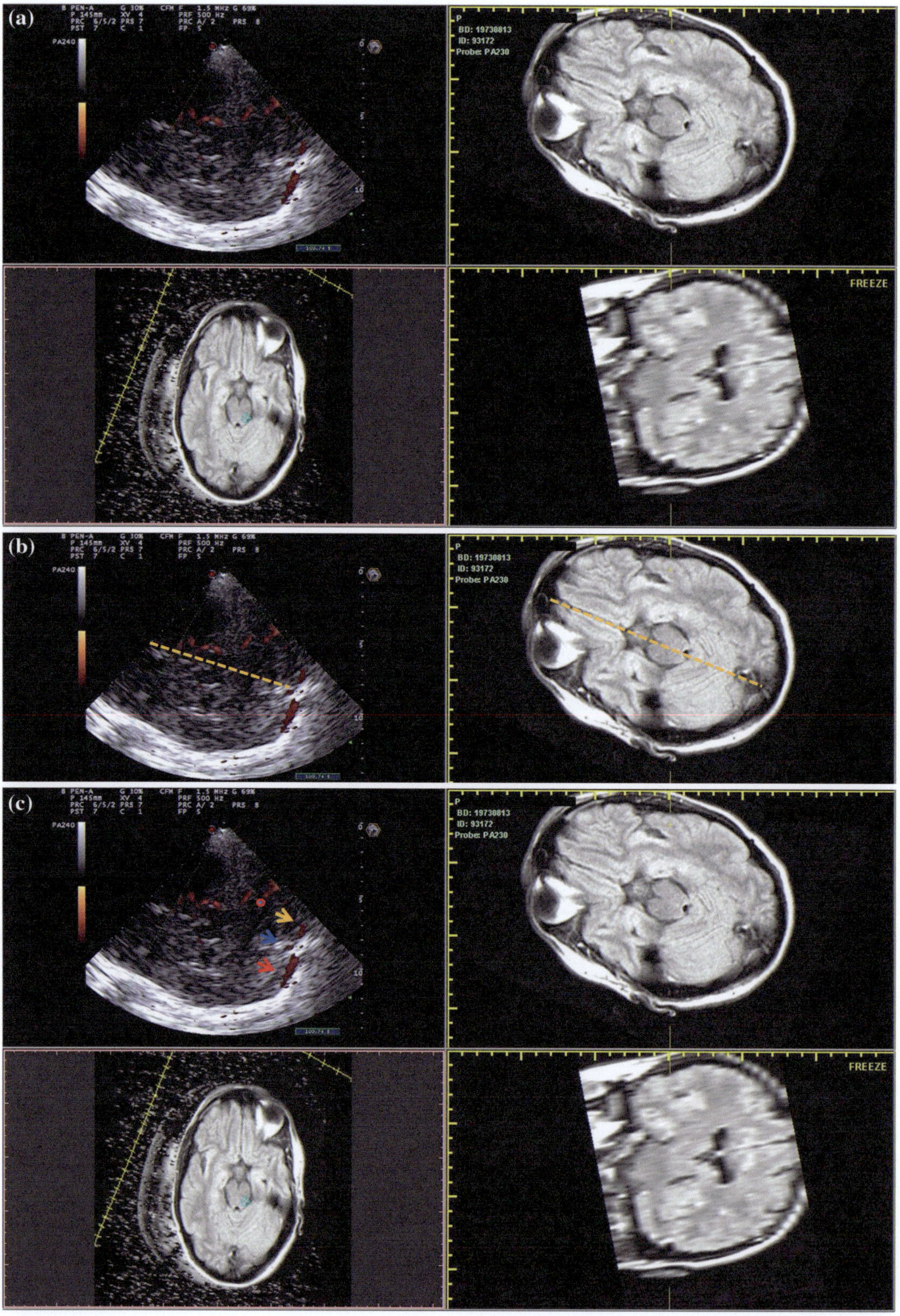
(a)
(b)
(c)
BD: 19730813
ID: 93172
Probe: PA230
FREEZE

Fig. 9.6 **a, b,** and **c** Oblique scan on the mesencephalic medium plane, with back angle (as evidenced by the angled position of the midline in (**b**). The third sector of this picture on the *left* highlights the upper portion of the posterior fossa, in power mode and Doppler mode, with the confluence of sinuses, the contralateral and ipsilateral TS, the mesencephalon in the middle third sector of the picture, with the venous structures "as a bridge" between the posterior fossa and the middle cranial fossa, the basal portion of the frontal lobes in the anterior third sector of the picture. In such a position, only the most basal portion of the polygon of Willis is insonable and in particular P1 and P2 PCA around the midbrain and the MCA origin. In (**b**), these anatomical structures are evidenced to make it easier to locate them; the red arrow indicates the contralateral TS, the yellow arrow marks the ipsilateral TS, the blue arrow shows the confluence of sinuses, while the red circle highlights the venous structures which are situated as a bridge between the posterior and the media cranial fossa

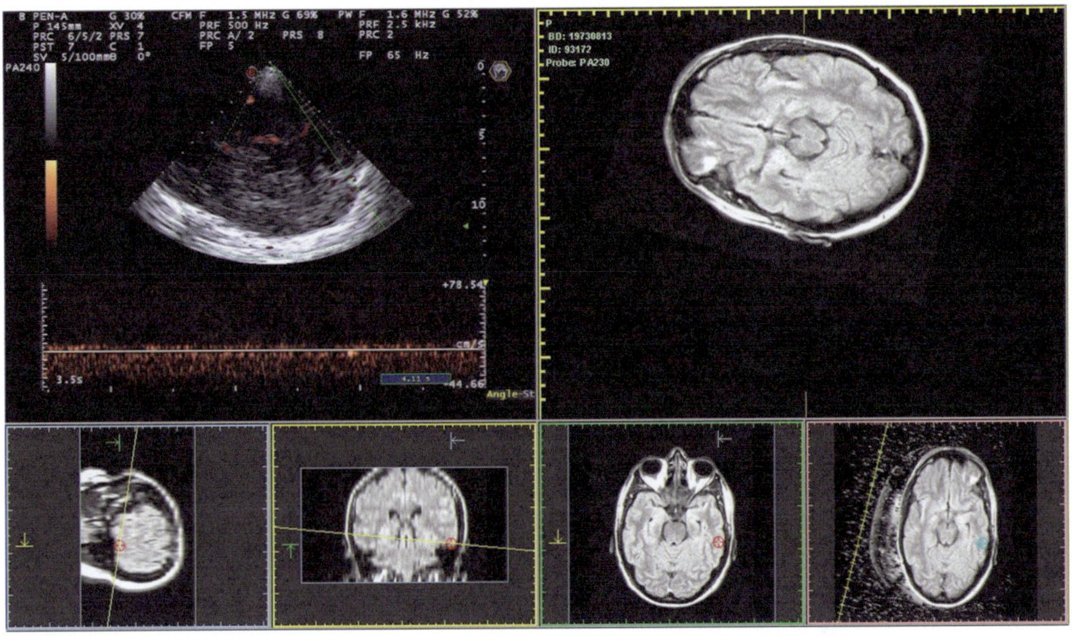

Fig. 9.7 In this figure and Fig. 9.8a, classical approach to the display of the contralateral TS is shown. The transducer is tilted obliquely, in a postero-superior way, thus allowing to insonate and to sample first the confluence of sinuses and the origin of the contralateral TS (Fig. 9.7), and then the next segment of the contralateral TS, without individuating the confluence of sinuses (Fig. 9.8). Comparing the two figures, you can observe the greater superior obliquity of the *left* portion of the image with the visualization of the more and more distal branches of the polygon of Willis. The scans on the virtual planes of MRI behave in a similar way, on the side

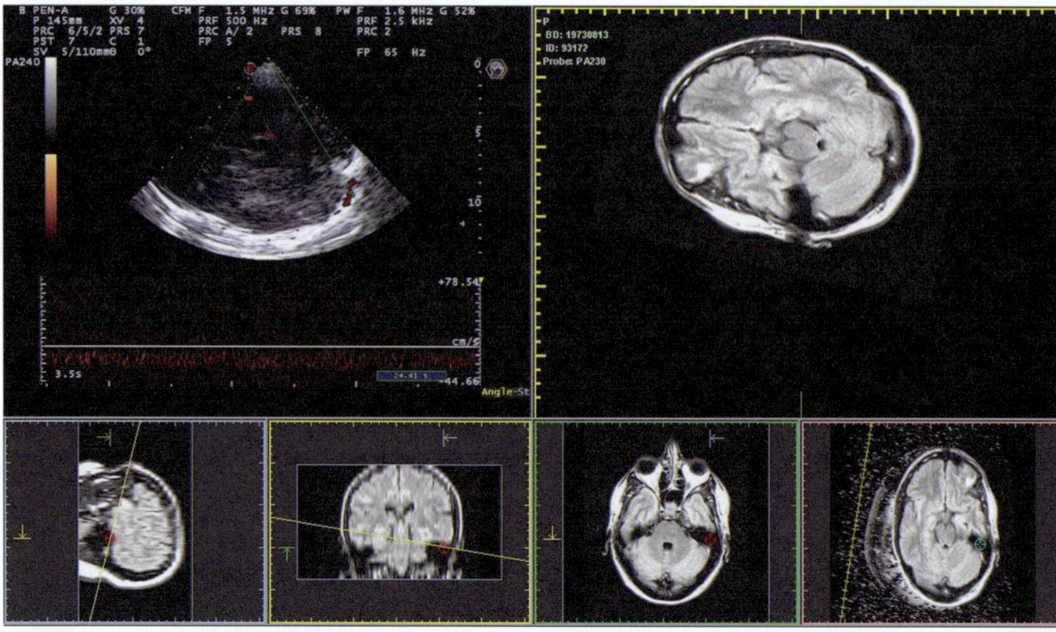

Fig. 9.8 In Fig. 9.7 and (**a**), classical approach to the display of the contralateral TS is shown. The transducer is tilted obliquely, in a postero-superior way, thus allowing to insonate and to sample first the confluence of sinuses and the origin of the contralateral TS (Fig. 9.7) and then the next segment of the contralateral TS, without individuating the confluence of sinuses (Fig. 9.8). Comparing the two figures, you can observe the greater superior obliquity of the left portion of the image with the visualization of the more and more distal branches of the Willis' circle. The scans on the virtual planes of MRI behave in a similar way, on the side

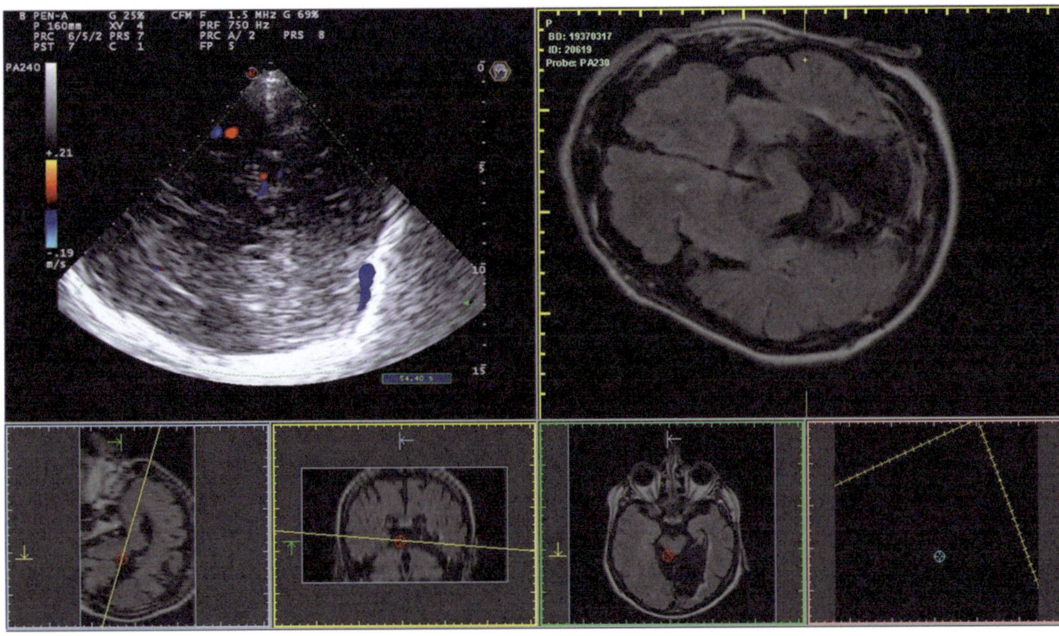

Fig. 9.9 It shows a further development of this different inclination of the probe. The anterior portion of the image is on an oblique plane passing through the mesencephalic–diencephalic plane, as can be identified both from the recognizable parenchymal structures and from the vascular information in color mode (MCA in the sylvian fissure and P3 PCA). The posterior portion is instead viewed obliquely postero-inferiorly at the limits of the posterior cranial fossa, with visualization of the contralateral TS coded in blue color and with the Doppler waveform away from the probe

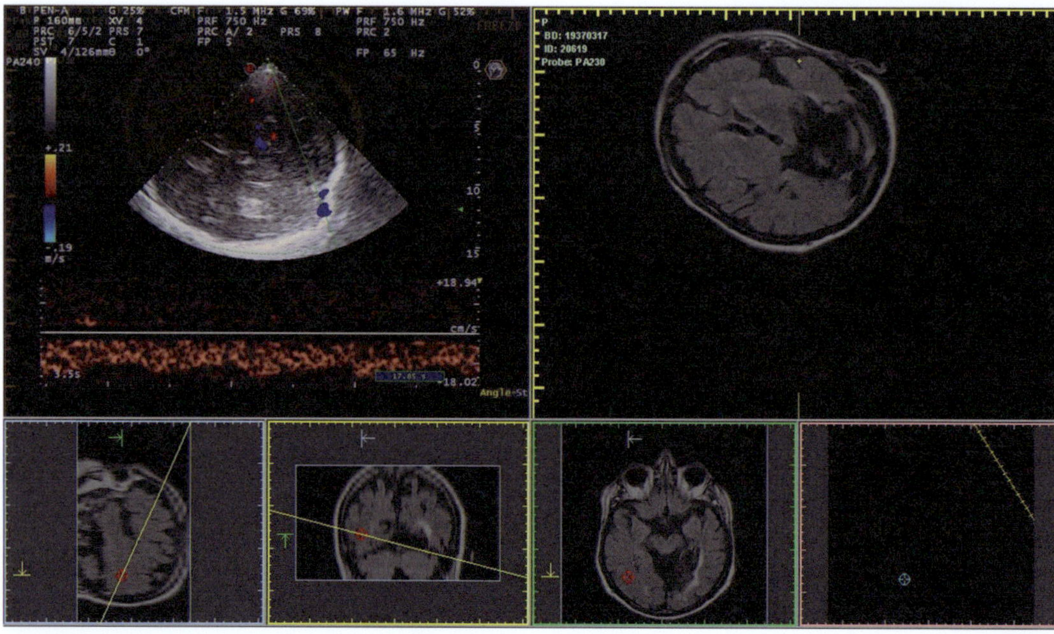

Fig. 9.10 By scanning in an even more tilted upward way, you switch directly to an oblique diencephalic plane (the third ventricle can be visualized, together with the frontal horns of the lateral ventricles). In this image, the structures of the posterior cranial fossa are no longer evident and the TS is not insonable. However, on the extreme rear of the midline, the posterior end of the SSS is displayed. It is visualized in blue color-coded and Doppler waveform away from the probe. Also in this case, it can be seen that there is a perfect match between the TCCS imaging and the corresponding MRI virtual plane, overlying it in the shadowing mode

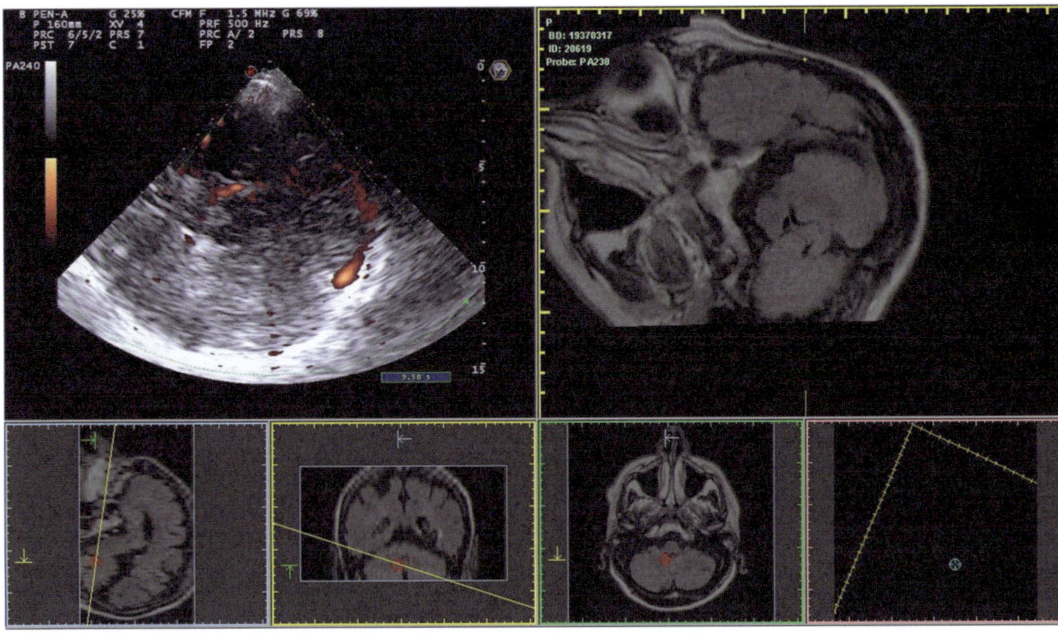

Fig. 9.11 A completely different access is made with an extreme back oblique scanning and a gradually *top*-to-*bottom* orientation, proceeding from the forehead to the occipital cerebellar. In this manner, exactly in the posterior cranial fossa, it is possible to view the ipsilateral TS adhering to the skull (power mode). The corresponding cerebral MRI image in virtual oblique plane confirms the anatomical counterpart with a higher spatial resolution technique and supplies a good intracranial anatomical reference. This scan, although less generally used, allows to evaluate almost the entire course of the ipsilateral TS, which is therefore differentiable in the medial, intermediate, and distal part [4, 5]

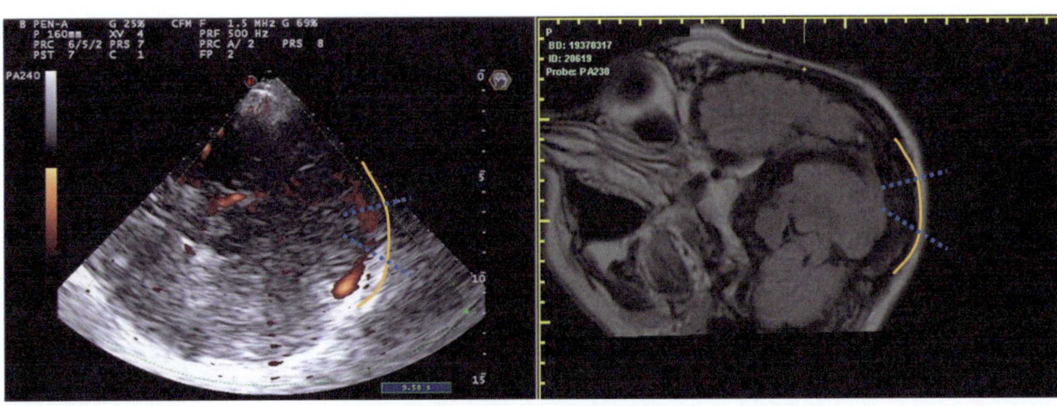

Fig. 9.12 A completely different access is made with an extreme back oblique scanning and a gradually *top*-to-*bottom* orientation, proceeding from the forehead to the occipital cerebellar. In this manner, exactly in the posterior cranial fossa, it is possible to view the ipsilateral TS adhering to the skull (power mode). The corresponding cerebral MRI image in virtual oblique plane confirms the anatomical counterpart with a higher spatial resolution technique and supplies a good intracranial anatomical reference. This scan, although less generally used, allows to evaluate almost the entire course of the ipsilateral TS, which is therefore differentiable in the medial, intermediate, and distal part [4, 5]

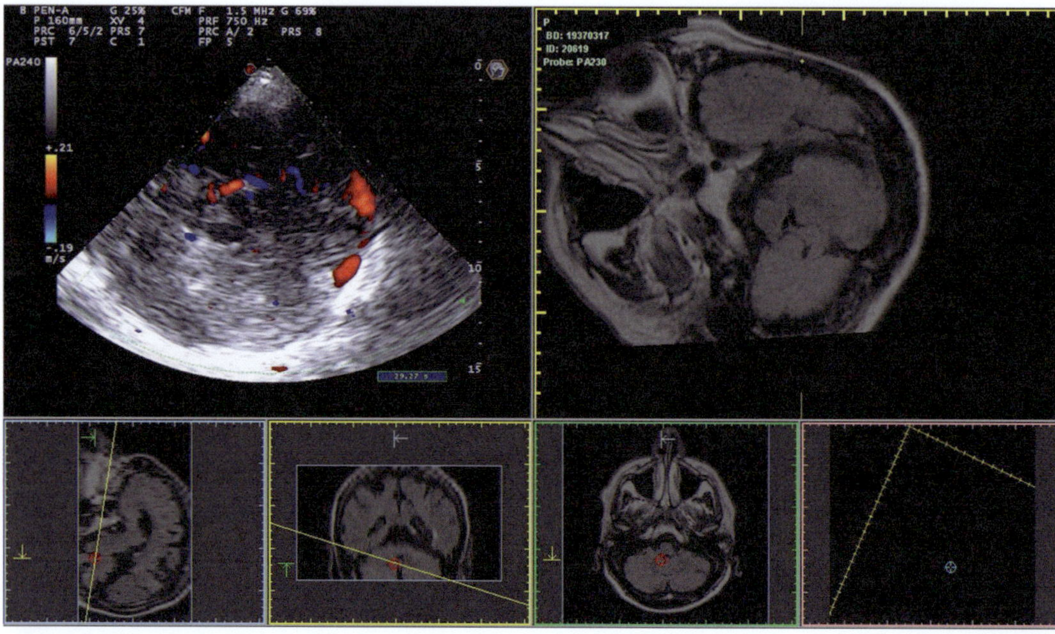

Fig. 9.13 The figure shows the same situation of the two previous ones (Figs. 9.11 and 9.12) and of Movie 9.3 but in color mode not in power mode: It is possible to appreciate the flow direction of both the arterial vascular structures (for example PCA) and the venous ones (ipsilateral TS). The ipsilateral TS appears to be adherent to the cranial theca and it is color-coded in red, that is with the flow direction approaching toward the probe

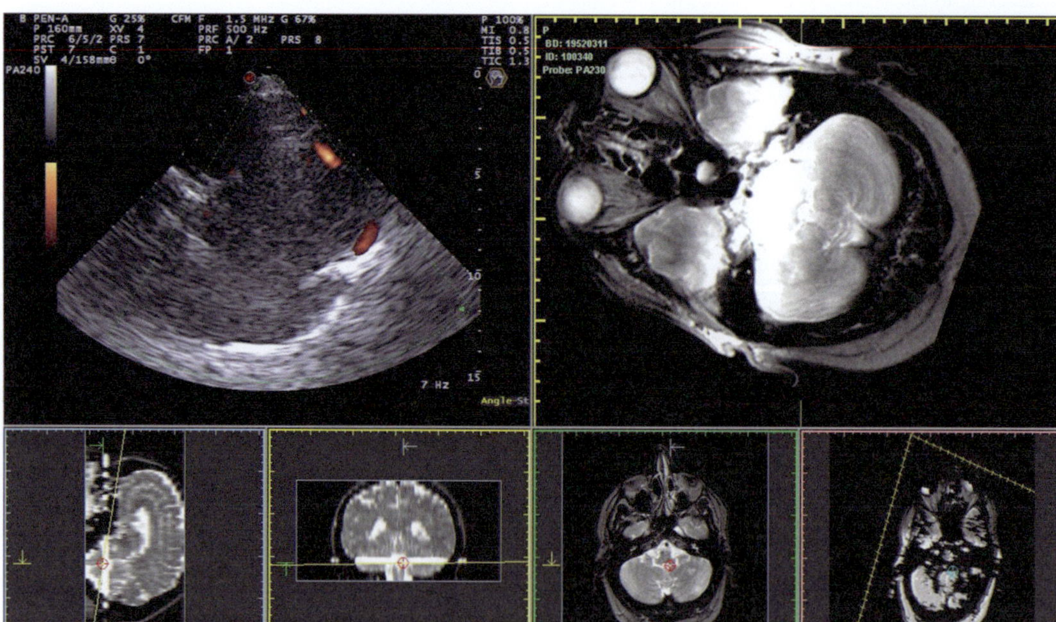

Fig. 9.14 The figure shows an example of insonation of the TS with an approach from the temporal window and an oblique orientation on the posterior fossa. This approach makes the main bony ultrasound landmarks (edge bone in the posterior fossa) available, with less parenchymal references. Furthermore, it allows to highlight (see power-mode signal) the ipsilateral TS in its proximal and distal portion. In addition, the corresponding MRI virtual scan clearly refers to the oblique plan orientation and to the location in the posterior fossa of the same TS

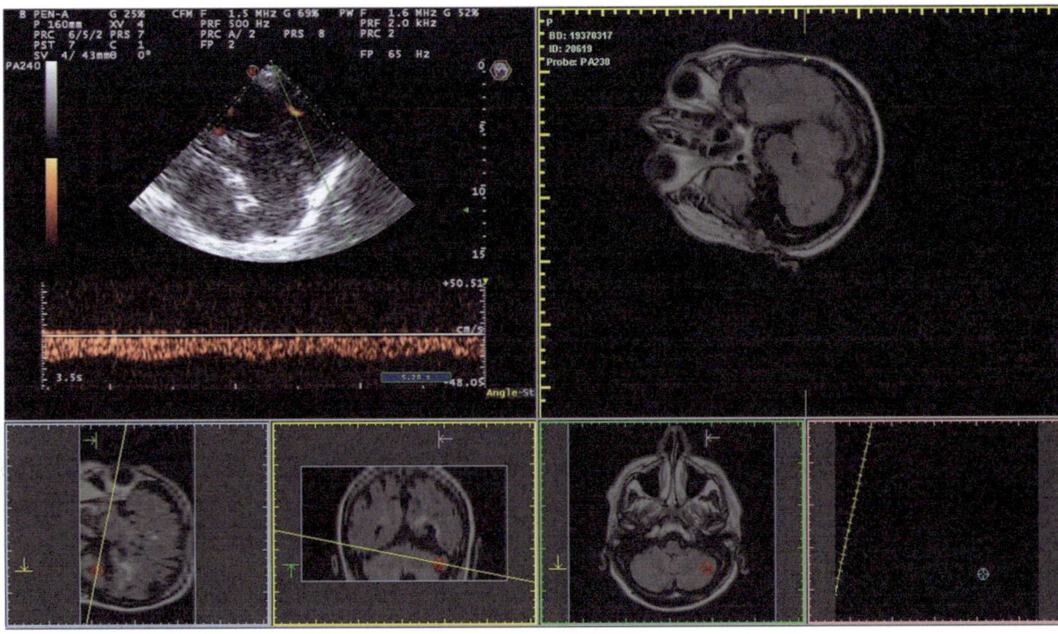

Fig. 9.15 In order to further confirm the correct identification of the insonated vessel, both the proximal and the distal ipsilateral TS signal flow can be sampled. The figure shows the Doppler waveform sampling of the ipsilateral TS in its distal segment, with direction away from the probe. This finding can besides be expected because of the curvature and the course of the vessel itself, which starts at the confluence of the SyS. The corresponding MRI image confirms the scanning plane and the anatomical landmarks

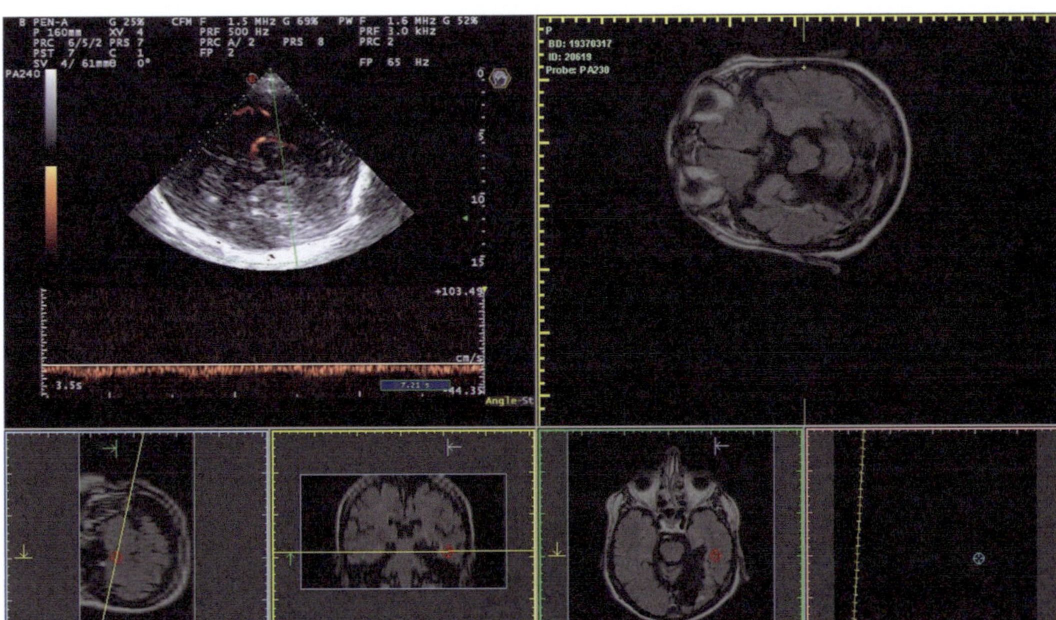

Fig. 9.16 The study with virtual navigator can be useful to define the anatomical–ultrasound relationships also when studying easily insonated vessels with established windows, such as the BVR in the post-communicating segment, around the cerebral peduncle and close to the P2-P3 PCA. In the figure, these anatomical relationships are well highlighted, together with the MRI corresponding scan, with conformity between the two methods of the scanning level of the mesencephalic section. The Doppler waveform of the post-peduncular BVR appears, as expected, with direction away from the probe

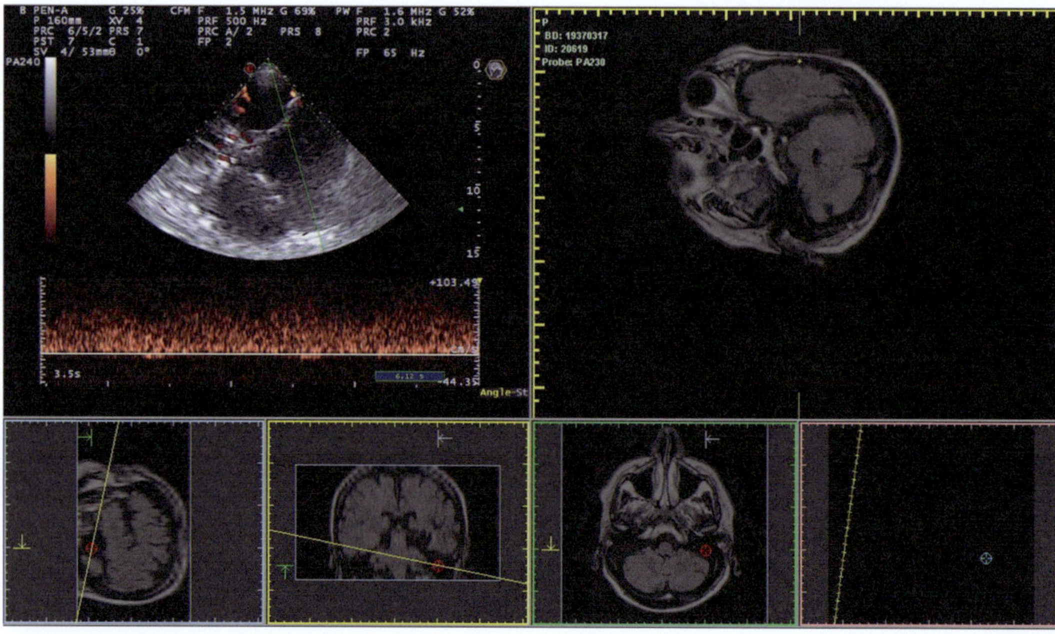

Fig. 9.17 Another blood vessel that can be explored in a less easily studied and standardized segment is the SPS. It represents an important route of connection between the system of the CS on one side and that of the TS-SyS on the other one. The picture, along the edge of the petrous bone, ipsilateral, shows the intermediate segment of the SPS with the Doppler waveform directed toward the probe (usually the sampling takes place in the medial segment and the direction of flow away from the probe is considered normal) and high speed (see Movie 9.7), with activation of the flow toward the TS-SyS in case of GV and SRS thrombosis

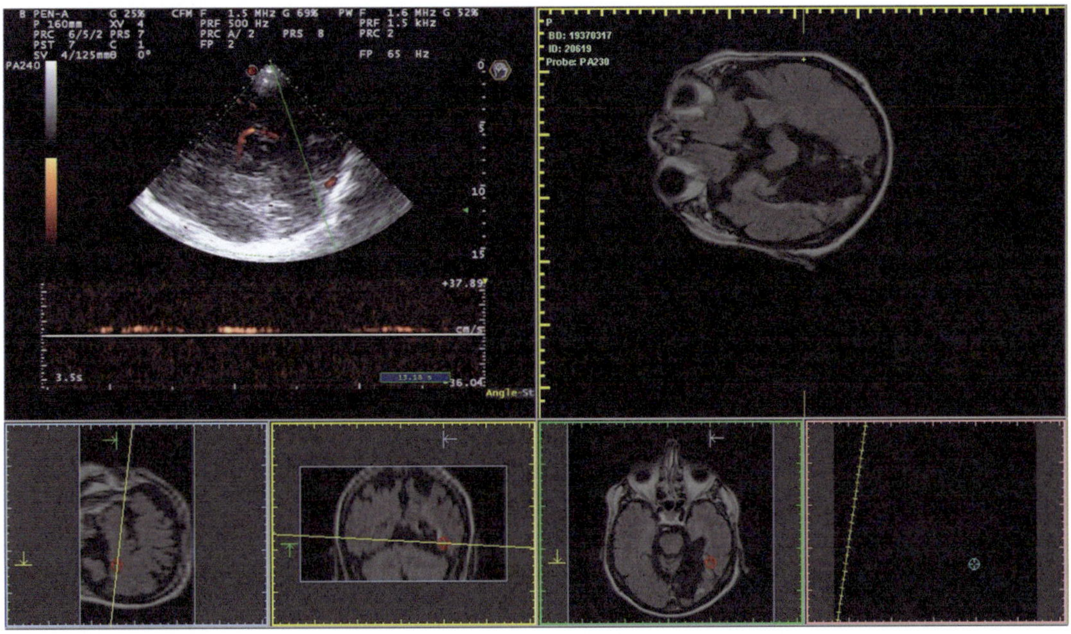

Fig. 9.18 The figure shows how the insonation of a hypoplastic TS, with contralateral approach, is facilitated by the image fusion method. In fact, it is possible to obtain the course of the vessel through the anatomical landmarks provided by the MRI corresponding scanning. This can be performed, also with low flow velocities, not always clearly identifiable even with the power mode. The characteristics and the Doppler waveform direction, basically monophasic and presenting direction toward the probe and low speeds, are consistent with hypoplasia, confirmed by MRI, in the absence of pathological situations

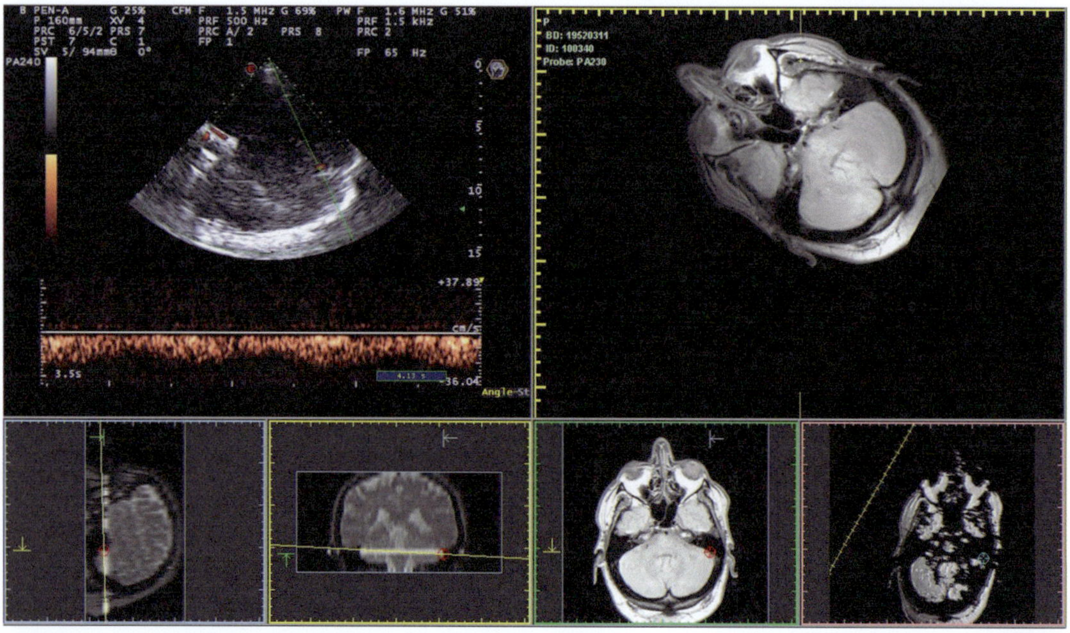

Fig. 9.19 The picture shows the insonation of a major venous sinus, collector of the deep venous system, that is the SRS, closely to its termination with access to the posterior fossa. It is performed in power mode and with the Doppler waveform away from the probe. Also in this case, it is possible to note the correspondence between the ultrasound image and cerebral MRI, as in Movie 9.11

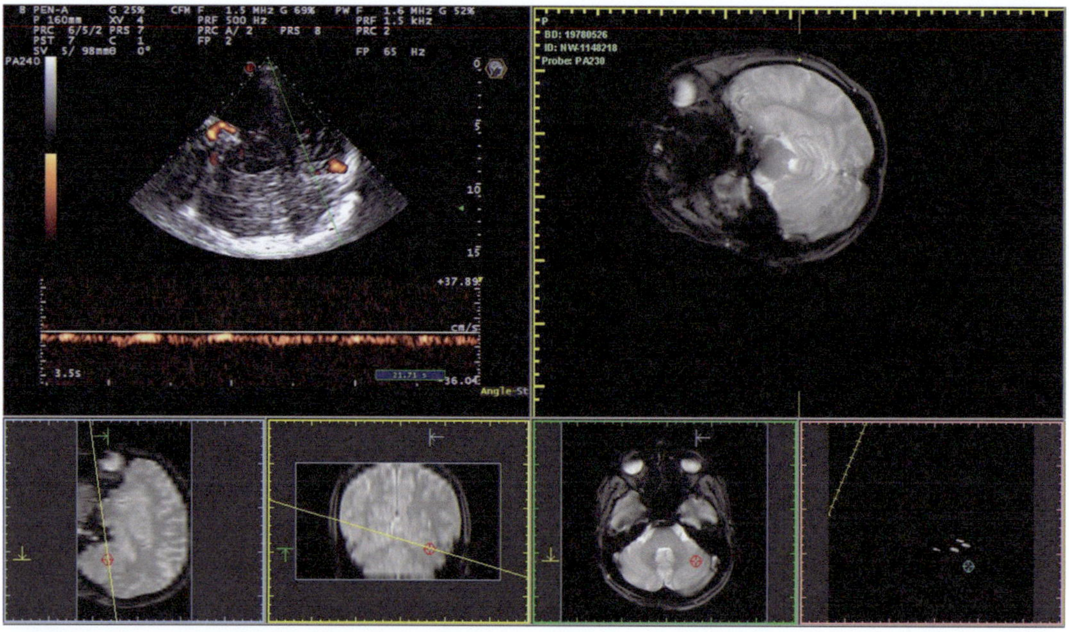

Fig. 9.20 SRS scanning from the posterior cranial fossa approach, similar but less oblique compared to the one shown in Fig. 9.19. The section of the mesencephalon comes clearly out both in the ultrasound and in the MRI planes. The Doppler waveform shows characteristics of pulsatility which are similar to the ones of Fig. 9.19 but with lower velocity

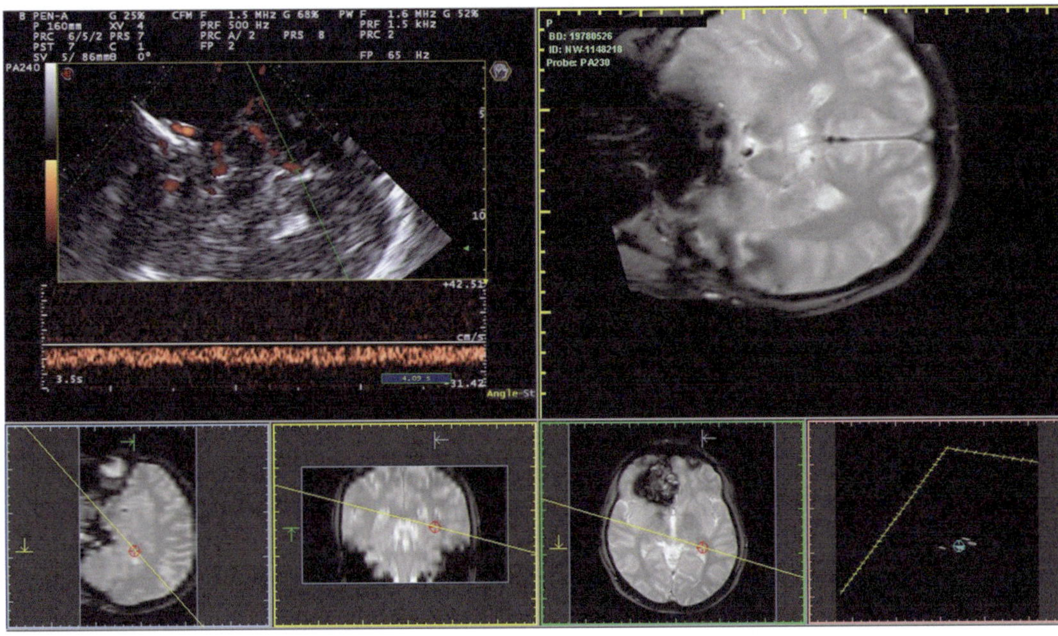

Fig. 9.21 Insonation of the GV, immediately after its origin from the confluence of the BVR and the ICV bilaterally, with magnified image (both MRI and ultrasound). It is possible to accurately display the first segment of the GV and the corresponding flow *waveform* on a high mesencephalic plan with the two imaging modalities. The dynamic assessment of the GV is shown in Movie 9.13. A voluminous frontal cavernous angioma represents a collateral landmark, detectable in brain MRI scans in the *bottom*

References

1. Nakano S, Yoshida M, Fujii K, Yorozuya K, Mouri Y, Kousaka J, Fukutomi T, Kimura J, Ishiguchi T, Ohno K, Mizumoto T, Harao M (2009) Fusion of MRI and sonography image for breast cancer evaluation using real-time virtual sonography with magnetic navigation: first experience. Jpn J Clin Oncol 39(9):552–559
2. Crocetti L, Lencioni R, DeBeni S, See TC, Della Pina C, Bartolozzi C (2008)Targeting liver lesions for radiofrequency ablation: an experimental feasibility study using a CT-US fusion imaging system. Invest Radiol 43(1):33–39
3. Minami Y, Chung H, Kudo M, Kitai S, Takahashi S, Inoue T, Ueshima K, Shiozaki H (2008) Radiofrequency ablation of hepatocellular carcinoma: value of virtual CT sonography with magnetic navigation, AJR 190(6):W335–W341
4. Zedde M, Malferrari G, De Berti G, Maggi M, Lodigiani L (2012) Virtual Navigator study: Subset of preliminary data about cerebral venous circulation. Perspect Med 1:385–389
5. Zedde M, Malferrari G, De Berti G, Maggi M (2012) Ipsilateral evaluation of the transverse sinus: transcranial color-coded sonography approach in comparison with magnetic resonance venography. Perspect Med 1:390–394

MIX
Papier aus verantwortungsvollen Quellen
Paper from responsible sources
FSC® C105338

If you have any concerns about our products,
you can contact us on
ProductSafety@springernature.com

In case Publisher is established outside the EU,
the EU authorized representative is:
Springer Nature Customer Service Center GmbH
Europaplatz 3, 69115 Heidelberg, Germany

Printed by Libri Plureos GmbH
in Hamburg, Germany